TRAUMA AND PHYSICAL HEALTH

UNDERSTANDING THE EFFECTS
OF EXTREME STRESS AND OF
PSYCHOLOGICAL HARM

Edited by Victoria L. Banyard,
Valerie J. Edwards, and
Kathleen A. Kendall-Tackett

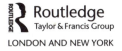

Routledge
Taylor & Francis Group

LONDON AND NEW YORK

First published 2009
by Routledge
2 Park Square, Milton Park, Abingdon, Oxon OX14 4RN

Simultaneously published in the USA and Canada
by Routledge
270 Madison Avenue, New York, NY 10016

Routledge is an imprint of the Taylor & Francis Group, an informa business

© 2009 selection and editorial matter, Victoria L. Banyard,
Valerie J. Edwards, and Kathleen A. Kendall-Tackett; individual chapters,
the contributors

Typeset in Frutiger by
Keystroke, 28 High Street, Tettenhall, Wolverhampton
Printed and bound in Great Britain by
CPI Antony Rowe, Chippenham, Wiltshire

British Library Cataloguing in Publication Data
A catalogue record for this book is available from the British Library

Library of Congress Cataloging-in-Publication Data
Trauma and physical health : understanding the effects of extreme stress and
of psychological harm / edited by Victoria L. Banyard,
Valerie J. Edwards, and Kathleen A. Kendall-Tackett.
p. ; cm.
Includes bibliographical references.
1. Post-traumatic stress disorder–Complications. 2. Psychic trauma–Complications.
3. Adult child abuse victims–Health and hygiene. I. Banyard, Victoria L.
II. Edwards, Valerie J. III. Kendall-Tackett, Kathleen A.
[DNLM: 1. Stress Disorders, Post-Traumatic–therapy. 2. Adult Survivors of Child
Abuse–psychology. 3. Domestic Violence–psychology. 4. Patient-Centered
Care–methods. 5. Primary Health Care. WM 170 T77725 2009]
RC552.P67T746 2009
616.85'21—dc22
2008026520

ISBN 10: 0–415–48078–7 (hbk)
ISBN 10: 0–415–48079–5 (pbk)
ISBN 10: 0–203–88501–5 (ebk)

ISBN 13: 978–0–415–48078–9 (hbk)
ISBN 13: 978–0–415–48079–6 (pbk)
ISBN 13: 978–0–203–88501–7 (ebk)

TRAUMA AND PHYSICAL HEALTH

Trauma research and clinical practice have taught us much about the widespread problems of child maltreatment, partner violence, and sexual assault. Numerous investigations have documented links between such trauma exposure and long-term negative mental health consequences. As we learn more about traumatic stress, however, increasing attention has been drawn to the less studied physical health effects of maltreatment and trauma.

Trauma and Physical Health describes both the negative physical health effects of victimization in childhood as well as exploring theoretical models that explain these links. By bringing together new and current studies on the relationship between trauma and physical health, this edited collection assesses the clinical implications of these links. At a time when the mental health field is becoming increasingly cognizant of the value of collaboration with professionals in the physical health arena, this book suggests ways in which clinicians can work with primary care professionals to better meet the needs of trauma survivors across the lifespan. A key focus of the text is to clarify the relationship between the current knowledge base in trauma and physical health and directions for future research in primary care health settings.

With contributors from a wide range of clinical and psychological disciplines, this book will be of interest to researchers, clinicians and professionals in the trauma field and to primary care professionals concerned with compassionate care for the traumatized.

Victoria L. Banyard is Full Professor of Psychology at the University of New Hampshire, USA.

Valerie J. Edwards is Research Psychologist at the Centers for Disease Control and Prevention, USA.

Kathleen A. Kendall-Tackett is Clinical Associate Professor of Pediatrics, Texas Tech University Health Sciences Center, USA.

Contents

Figure and tables

Contributors

Bruce Ambuel, PhD, is Associate Professor of Family and Community Medicine at the Medical College of Wisconsin. He is an expert in health psychology, community research and action. Dr. Ambuel's research and advocacy focus on primary and secondary prevention of intimate partner violence (IPV) through health care systems, and developing community partnerships to promote health in underserved, marginalized communities. He leads 2 grants, *Health Care Can Change from Within: A Sustainable Model of Intimate Partner Violence Prevention in Health Care*, and a grant implementing IPV education for medical students.

Victoria L. Banyard, PhD, is Full Professor in the Department of Psychology at the University of New Hampshire. She received her doctorate in clinical psychology with a certificate in Women's Studies from the University of Michigan. She has completed postdoctoral research and clinical training at the Family Research Lab at UNH and the Trauma Center in Boston. She conducts research on the long-term consequences of trauma and interpersonal violence including factors related to resilience and recovery. She was the principal investigator on a study examining the efficacy of a college rape prevention program and has begun a program of research with several colleagues on broader community approaches to sexual and intimate partner violence prevention.

Kiara Cromer, MS, is a doctoral candidate in Clinical Psychology at Florida State University. She graduated from Whitworth College with a Bachelor of Science degree in Biochemistry. After graduation, she accepted a position at the Laboratory of Clinical Science within the National Institute of Mental Health investigating the neurobiology of neuropsychiatric disorders, using molecular, neurochemical and genetic techniques. Kiara's primary research interests lie in understanding the etiology, comorbidity, and maintenance of obsessive-compulsive disorder, focusing on risk factors and vulnerability mechanisms. She is particularly interested in linking behavior with underlying biological factors such as genetics, and examining the role that stress plays in the pathogenesis of psychiatric disorders. She also has been conducting epidemiological research in the area of childhood abuse, specifically the role stress plays in influencing genetic and environmental risk factors for health problems among individuals who experienced childhood abuse.

Stephanie Dallam, RN, MS, is a doctoral candidate at the University of Kansas. She also is Research Associate for the Leadership Council on Child Abuse and Interpersonal Violence. Prior to this, she worked as Nurse Practitioner in Pediatric Trauma and Surgery at the University of Missouri-Columbia. She has written numerous articles and book chapters on issues related to the heath effects of childhood maltreatment and presents regularly at national conferences.

Valerie J. Edwards, PhD, is Research Psychologist at the U.S. Centers for Disease Control and Prevention. For the past ten years, she has been a member of the Adverse Childhood Experiences study team.

Ulrich Tiber Egle, MD, is Medical Director of the Psychosomatic Clinic Kinzigtal, and Professor of Psychosomatic Medicine and Psychotherapy, Johannes Gutenberg University,

Mainz, Germany. He is past president of the German College for Psychosomatic Medicine (DKPM) and president of the Interdisciplinary Society for Psychosomatic Pain Therapy (IGPS). He has written some 200 articles and edited three books (in German) on the psychobiological aspects of chronic pain, somatoform disorders, and the long-term psychological and physical consequences of childhood trauma.

Cynthia Good Mojab, MS, IBCLC, RLC, CATSM, is Director of LifeCircle Counseling and Consulting in Hillsboro, Oregon. As a researcher, clinical counselor, and International Board Certified Lactation Consultant, she has a special interest in helping women recover from traumatic events related to pregnancy loss, birth, and infant death, as well as in the development of evidence-based approaches to the delivery of breastfeeding-compatible mental health care. She is a member of the American Academy of Experts in Traumatic Stress and of the National Center for Crisis Management and is Certified in Acute Traumatic Stress Management. Ms. Good Mojab is the founder of LactPsych, an international group of professionals working in the emerging field of lactational psychology. She formerly served as Research Associate at La Leche League International and was on the faculty of Parkland College. She has authored and contributed to numerous publications related to breastfeeding, culture, and psychology.

L. Kevin Hamberger, PhD, is Professor of Family and Community Medicine at the Medical College of Wisconsin and Co-Chair of the Wisconsin Governor's Council for Domestic Abuse. He has served as a consultant to the National Institutes of Health, National Institute of Mental Health, the National Institute of Justice, the Department of Defense, and the Family Violence Prevention Fund. He is on the editorial boards of six scholarly journals and has published 96 articles and chapters, and six books, including *Violence Issues for Health Care Educators and Providers* (The Haworth Press) and *Domestic*

Violence Screening in Medical and Mental Healthcare Settings with Dr. Mary Beth Phelan (Springer).

Annya Hernandez, MS, was born to Cuban political exiles in Santurce, Puerto Rico, grew up in Miami, Florida, and graduated from Harvard University with honors in the field of psychology. She is presently completing her doctorate in Clinical Psychology from Florida State University. She conducts research in the area of psychiatric epidemiology, and her research specialty is on the effects of culture on psychiatric and health problems among Hispanic population residing in the United States.

Kathleen A. Kendall-Tackett, PhD, IBCLC is Health Psychologist and an International Board Certified Lactation Consultant. She is Clinical Associate Professor of Pediatrics at Texas Tech University Health Sciences Center and Acquisitions Editor for Hale Publishing. Dr. Kendall-Tackett is a Fellow of the American Psychological Association in both the Divisions of Health and Trauma Psychology. She is Editor of *Family and Intimate Partner Violence Quarterly*, Associate Editor of the American Psychological Association's journal, *Psychological Trauma*, and serves on the editorial boards of four other journals in family violence and perinatal health. Dr. Kendall-Tackett is author of more than 180 journal articles, book chapters and other publications, and author or editor of 17 books in the fields of trauma, women's health, interpersonal violence, and depression. She is a founding member of the American Psychological Association's Division of Trauma Psychology, and currently serves as Division Secretary

Gerri C. Lasiuk, RN, MN, PhD, CMHPN(C) is Assistant Professor with the Faculty of Nursing, University of Alberta, Canada. Dr. Lasiuk's clinical and research interests include the health effects of childhood adversity, the experience of pregnancy and birthing among women with histories of child sexual abuse, and the sensitive health care of men and women who were abused in childhood.

Patrick Luyten, PhD, is Assistant Professor at the Department of Psychology, University of Leuven (Belgium). His main research interest focuses on the role of personality, stress and interpersonal processes in depression, chronic fatigue syndrome and fibromyalgia. He is currently also involved in studies on the mentalization-based treatment of patients with borderline personality disorder. He is a visiting professor at the Department of Psychology, University College London, London (UK), a visiting research scholar at the Yale Child Study Center, New Haven (USA), and member of the Research Advisory Board and the Conceptual and Empirical Research Committee of the International Psychoanalytical Association (IPA).

Mary Beth Phelan, MD, is Associate Professor of Emergency Medicine in the Department of Emergency Medicine, and an affiliate faculty member of the Injury Research Center at the Medical College of Wisconsin. Dr. Phelan's areas of interest include the health consequences of intimate partner violence, injury prevention and intimate partner violence education for health care providers. She has collaborated with researchers to determine the impact of intimate partner violence on women and men seeking emergency medical treatment. Dr. Phelan has co-authored the book *Domestic Violence Screening in Medical and Mental Healthcare Settings* (Springer).

Natalie Sachs-Ericsson, PhD, Clinical Psychologist, is on the faculty in the Department of Psychology at Florida State University. Her research expertise is in psychiatric and health epidemiology, and she has published extensively (over 50 peer reviewed journal articles and several book chapters) on genetic, environmental, family, and social influences in the development of psychiatric and health problems, including the influence of childhood abuse experiences on health and psychiatric disorders.

Candice L. Schachter, PT, PhD, Adjunct Professor, School of Physical Therapy, University of Saskatchewan, is the principal investigator of the multi-phased, multidisciplinary Sensitive Practice Research Project that has sought to facilitate better health care experiences for adult survivors of childhood sexual abuse. She has lectured on Sensitive Practice internationally. Her research team has just completed the gender inclusive, second edition of the *Handbook of Sensitive Practice: Lessons from Adult Survivors of Childhood Sexual Abuse* (Public Health Agency of Canada).

Carol A. Stalker, PhD, RSW, Professor, Faculty of Social Work, Wilfrid Laurier University, has worked therapeutically with survivors of child sexual abuse (CSA) in mental health settings and in private practice. She teaches clinical social work courses and conducts research to increase understanding of the impact of CSA and to evaluate the effectiveness of mental health interventions with survivors

Eli Teram, PhD, Professor, Faculty of Social Work, Wilfrid Laurier University, is currently involved in research projects related to social work ethics, sensitive health practice, youth resilience and mergers between not-for-profit organizations.

Boudewijn Van Houdenhove, MD, is Clinical Head of the Department of Liaison Psychiatry, University Hospitals Leuven, and Professor of Medical and Health Psychology, Faculty of Medicine, University of Leuven, Belgium. He has been clinically and scientifically involved in the field of psychosomatic medicine for more than 35 years, with a special interest in stress-related physical disorders, particularly chronic pain and fatigue. His research focuses on the relations between these disorders and early-life stress, personality and lifestyle, and applies to psychological as well as neurobiological aspects. His publications include some 200 articles and 7 books (in Dutch) on psychosomatics and liaison psychiatry.

Marie Wolff, PhD, is Associate Professor in the Department of Family and Community Medicine at the Medical College of Wisconsin. Dr. Wolff has a research and programmatic emphasis on community academic partnerships to improve health.

Dr. Wolff was Project Director of a three year Health Resources and Services Administration (HRSA) Graduate Medical Education grant to strengthen the community health curriculum in four Family Medicine residency programs with a primary focus on the prevention of intimate partner violence. She has also developed and pilot tested an Objective Structured Clinical Exam (OSCE) to assess Family, Emergency Medicine and Pediatric residents on the skills necessary to competently conduct primary and secondary prevention of intimate partner violence.

Introduction to trauma and physical health

A framework and introduction to integrating trauma practice into primary care

Victoria L. Banyard, Kathleen A. Kendall-Tackett and Valerie J. Edwards

RESEARCH AND CLINICAL PRACTICE with trauma survivors have taught us much about the widespread problems of child maltreatment, partner violence, and sexual assault. Numerous investigations have documented links between such trauma exposure and long-term negative mental health consequences. We have also identified risk and protective factors for more resilient functioning. As we learn more about the psychobiology of traumatic stress, however, increasing attention has been drawn to understanding physical health effects of maltreatment and trauma (e.g., Kendall-Tackett, 2003). In a recent book reviewing this research on the link between childhood abuse and adult health problems, Kendall-Tackett (2003) describes a model that explains these links. She points out that much more needs to be learned given that the majority of research on trauma and maltreatment has focused on mental health symptoms.

The appearance of growing numbers of empirical articles addressing trauma and physical health coincides with an increasing interest in collaborating with professionals in medicine and nursing. For example, Frank *et al.* (2004), in *Primary care psychology*, outline important roles for mental health clinicians in primary care settings. Several sections of the book describe how trauma both directly and indirectly impacts physical health through its association with psychological distress. This book suggests ways in which clinicians with expertise in trauma treatment may partner in important ways with primary care professionals to better meet the needs of trauma survivors across the lifespan. Indeed, a recent article in *Pediatrics* (Borowsky *et al.*, 2004) presents research on how primary care physicians can help prevent future violence and aggression when they screen for violence among children.

But where are we to go from here? Merrill and colleagues (2001, pp. 992–993) describe a useful framework for examining progress in research. Although their model focuses specifically on the field of child sexual abuse, it has applications as an organizing frame for the field of trauma, physical health, and primary care intervention. They describe three levels of research that need to occur for a field to move forward. Contributors to this volume have written chapters that fall within each of these levels. These are described below.

"First-generation" research aims to establish clear links between trauma and its effects across a wide variety of samples, for a variety of outcomes. This has been an important focus of research on trauma and physical health to date given that most early research on the short- and long-term consequences of abuse focused almost exclusively on mental health outcomes. Most of the chapters that follow review the extensive and growing literature that establishes the negative impact of trauma on health symptoms and behaviors across the lifespan. Vanhoudenhove *et al.*, Sachs-Ericsson *et al.*, and Good Mojab continue this line of work in their explorations of links between trauma and health outcomes that have received relatively less attention, including chronic fatigue and pain, and postpartum health.

"Second-generation" studies, according to Merrill *et al.*, are those that move beyond comparisons of victims and non-victims to within-group analyses examining factors which moderate the degree of effects that trauma has on outcomes. In their particular review of research on child sexual abuse, they discuss variations in characteristics of the abuse that may impact patterns of distress and resilience among groups of survivors. Chapters in this volume point to ways in which more work is needed in this area for understanding trauma and physical health. In particular, Banyard points to ways in which gender has been an understudied aspect of this topic and presents implications for both future research and practice. Further, the chapters in the current book demonstrate the impact of a wide array of trauma experiences on physical health, rather than focusing exclusively on child maltreatment as Merrill *et al.* do, or as was more common in early inquiry into links between trauma and physical health. This work encourages us to ask questions about how different types of trauma may be associated with different health outcomes and the need for different types of intervention and prevention efforts.

Finally, Merrill *et al.* describe "third-generation studies," which aim to illustrate and gather evidence for processes through which trauma impacts outcomes. It allows us to ask questions about what variables may explain the powerful links we find between trauma exposure and physical health symptoms. Such research holds the key to important information for the design of effective intervention efforts. The chapter by Kendall-Tackett provides a review of two newly hypothesized mediating mechanisms in need of future study: self-efficacy and sleep deprivation. The links from such discussions to practice are highlighted in each chapter but particularly by Dallam, Stalker, and Hamberger, who describe guidelines for specific practices within primary care settings that may address such mediating processes and help interrupt the link between trauma exposure and negative physical health.

Indeed, a key aim of the current volume is to make clear the relationship between both what the field currently knows about trauma and physical health, and directions for future research as they may be applied to work within primary care health settings. The chapters ground us in a review of what is known while then asking the next set of questions and discussing real-world implications that the answers may hold.

REFERENCES

Borowsky, I.W., Mozayeny, S., Stuenkey, K., and Ireland, M. (2004). Effects of a primary care-based intervention on violent behavior and injury in children. *Pediatrics, 114*, 392–399.

Frank, R.G., McDaniel, S.H., Bray, J.H., and Heldring, M. (2004). *Primary care psychology*. Washington, DC: American Psychological Association.

Kendall-Tackett, K. (2003). *Treating the lifetime health effects of childhood victimization*. Kingston, NJ: Civic Research Institute.

Merrill, L.L., Thomsen, C.J., Sinclair, B.B., Gold, S.R., and Milner, J.S. (2001). Predicting the impact of child sexual abuse on women: The role of abuse severity, parental support, and coping strategies. *Journal of Consulting and Clinical Psychology, 69*, 992–1006.

The views expressed in this introduction are those of the author(s) and do not necessarily represent the official position of the Centers for Disease Control and Prevention.

1

The association between childhood abuse, health and pain-related problems, and the role of psychiatric disorders and current life stress

Natalie Sachs-Ericsson, Kiara Cromer, Annya Hernandez, and Kathleen A. Kendall-Tackett

---

A GROWING BODY of literature has established an association between childhood abuse and adult health problems. In the current chapter we review the literature which has generally shown an association between childhood abuse (physical and/or sexual) and subsequent health problems, as well as increased pain reports in association with health problems. We will also discuss our research based on the National Comorbidity Survey (NCS), a representative sample of men and women aged 15 to 54 from the US population. Using these data, we have shown that health problems are distinctly increased in individuals who have experienced childhood sexual or physical abuse, that individuals who experienced childhood abuse report more pain in association with their health problems, and that current life stressors moderate the relationship between abuse and health such that the presence of stress doubles the effect of childhood abuse on health problems. We also discuss the influence of psychiatric disorders on the relationship between abuse and health problems.

We review theories underlying the association between childhood abuse and health functioning, including how early abuse may affect brain functioning to increase vulnerability to stress and decrease immune functioning. We discuss how childhood abuse is related to risky behaviors that are detrimental to health. Further, we discuss why there may be an association between childhood abuse and psychiatric disorders which in turn influences health and pain-related problems. Treatment recommendations are reviewed.

CHILDHOOD ABUSE AND MEDICAL PROBLEMS IN CLINICAL SAMPLES

Early studies, predominately of clinical samples of women, have found that medical problems are often overrepresented among individuals who have experienced childhood sexual abuse or childhood physical abuse (Sachs-Ericsson *et al.*, 2005). For example, studies have found sexual and physical abuse to be associated with diabetes (Kendall-Tackett and Marshall, 1999), gastrointestinal problems (Drossman *et al.*, 1995), obesity (Williamson *et al.*, 2002), and irritable bowel disease (Talley *et al.*, 1995).

Many of these earlier studies have been based on patients seeking medical treatment. Childhood abuse has been found to be associated with increased use of health services (Biggs *et al.*, 2003; Finestone *et al.*, 2000) and, thus, firm conclusions regarding the relationship between abuse and health cannot be based on clinical samples alone. However, studies of representative community population samples have generally confirmed the association between childhood abuse and health observed in clinical samples.

EPIDEMIOLOGICAL STUDIES OF ABUSE AND MEDICAL PROBLEMS

In a series of epidemiological investigations, Golding and colleagues consistently found a relationship between lifetime sexual abuse (occurring either in childhood or adulthood) and measures of overall health (Golding, 1994, 2003; Golding et al., 1997). Using data from a large, nationally representative sample of men and women, researchers (Thompson et al., 2004) found that physical abuse in childhood was related to health problems in adulthood for the sample as a whole.

Other studies have found increased rates of specific health problems among individuals with abuse histories. Specific health problems, such as gynecological problems, headaches, diabetes, arthritis, breast cancer for women (Golding, 1994, 1999; Golding et al., 1998; Stein and Barrett-Connor, 2000) and thyroid disease for men (Stein and Barrett-Connor, 2000) are higher for those who experienced sexual abuse in their lifetime. Further, childhood sexual abuse has been found to be associated with chronic fatigue, bladder problems, asthma, and heart problems (Dong et al., 2004; Romans et al., 2002). In her review of the literature, Leserman (2005) concluded that childhood sexual abuse appears to be related to a greater likelihood of headache, gastrointestinal, and gynecological problems. Childhood physical abuse has also been found to be associated with increased risk of specific health problems in adulthood. For example, both childhood sexual and physical abuse was found to be associated with ischemic heart disease (Dong et al., 2004). Further, in a national representative epidemiological survey of adults, an association between childhood physical abuse and increased odds of gastrointestinal problems and migraine headaches were found (Goodwin et al., 2003).

In our studies using a population sample from the National Comorbidity Survey (NCS; Sachs-Ericsson et al., 2005), we found childhood sexual and physical abuse to be associated with the one-year prevalence of serious health problems for both men and women, even after controlling for an array of family-of-origin problems (e.g., family-of-origin income, early parental loss, and parental psychiatric problems), as well as controlling for participants' psychiatric problems. Specifically, we found that individuals who had been physically abused as children (controlling for the effects of sexual abuse and other covariates) were more than twice as likely as those who had not been physically abused to have a serious health problem. In addition, those who had been sexually abused (controlling for the effects of physical abuse) were almost one-and-a-half times as likely to have a current serious health problem compared to those who had not been sexually abused.

In further analyses of the data, we found that childhood physical and sexual abuse was associated with increased prevalence of a number of specific medical problems. After controlling for the influence of family-of-origin variables and participants' current psychiatric diagnoses, the relationship between childhood abuse and several health problems remained significant including blindness or deafness; heart problems; and lupus, thyroid, or autoimmune problems (Cromer and Sachs-Ericsson, 2006).

CHILDHOOD ABUSE AND PAIN

Researchers from a wide range of medical specialties have noted that a relatively high percentage of patients with painful medical conditions and chronic pain have a history of childhood physical or sexual abuse (Kendall-Tackett, 2001). Specifically, clinical studies have found a higher proportion of child abuse survivors among patients with generalized pain (Finestone *et al.*, 2000; Green *et al.*, 2001; Kendall-Tackett, 2001; Kendall-Tackett *et al.*, 2003), pelvic pain and vulvodynia (Harlow and Stewart, 2005; Lampe *et al.*, 2003; Latthe *et al.*, 2006), fibromyalgia (Boisset-Pioro *et al.*, 1995), chronic musculoskeletal pain (Kopec and Sayre, 2004), headache (Golding, 1999), and irritable bowel syndrome and gastrointestinal illnesses (Drossman *et al.*, 2000; Leserman *et al.*, 1996; Talley *et al.*, 1995).

Epidemiological and case-controlled studies have generally supported findings from medically based samples. Epidemiological studies have documented that several painful medical conditions (e.g., painful gynecological problems, headaches, arthritis, musculature pain, tender-point pain, back pain, and generally distressing physical symptoms) are overrepresented in individuals with abuse histories (Golding, 1994, 1999; Goodwin et al., 2003; Linton, 2002; McBeth et al., 1999; Romans et al., 2002).

However, Raphael and colleagues have argued that the data are not altogether consistent. In their review of the literature of case-controlled and epidemiological studies, Raphael and colleagues (Raphael et al., 2004) point out that only cross-sectional studies with relatively large samples have consistently found a relationship between childhood abuse and painful medical conditions (i.e., pain associated with chronic pelvic pain, headache, back or neck pain, and general widespread pain). Specifically, five out of six cross-sectional studies (including those involving community and primary care samples) reported higher rates of pain associated with childhood sexual abuse (Bendixen et al., 1994; Jamieson and Steege, 1997; Linton, 1997; Newman et al., 2000; Romans et al., 2002). For two cross-sectional studies on childhood physical abuse and pain (Goodwin et al., 2003; Romans et al., 2002), only one found an association.

In a longitudinal study (based on participants' retrospective reports of abuse), Linton and colleagues (Linton, 2002) found that among participants with no pain at baseline, childhood abuse was associated with an increased occurrence of new episodes of back pain one year later. However, for those already reporting back pain at baseline, no association between childhood sexual or physical abuse and pain at follow-up was shown (Linton, 2002).

In another study, prospective findings (based on documented abuse cases in childhood) differed from retrospective findings (based on self-report in adulthood) for the same sample (Raphael et al., 2001). In this study, documented cases of sexually and physically abused and neglected children were matched with non-abused children. Participants were followed prospectively and in adulthood were asked to report retrospectively about childhood abuse experiences. Interestingly, almost half (49 percent) of the "non-abused" matched control group retrospectively reported childhood abuse experiences. Since the control group also had high numbers of abuse survivors, it is not surprising that there would be no difference between groups on rates of chronic pain syndromes. However, the retrospective data from these participants were consistent with previous studies finding an association between childhood abuse and pain.

DIFFERENCES DUE TO MEDICAL CONDITIONS

Differences in studies' findings may reflect, in part, which medical conditions are being identified. Examining differences in the population between abused and non-abused participants for painful conditions that have relatively low base rates are less likely to show significant results than disorders that are more prevalent. In this regard, most of the studies have been limited to a specific type of painful medical condition (e.g., headache, back pain, musculoskeletal pain (Raphael *et al.*, 2004)). Studies have commonly not identified the potential range of medical problems that may have been experienced by the participant, and the level of pain experienced in relation to current health problems. This may have attenuated the true relationship between childhood abuse and painful medical conditions.

In our research with the NCS sample, we examined a wide range of medical problems and the degree of reported pain associated with each of these conditions, and compared individuals with a history of childhood abuse (sexual and physical) to those with no abuse history. We found that individuals who experienced abuse reported more pain in relation to their current health problems than those without abuse experiences (Sachs-Ericsson *et al.*, 2007).

ADDITIVE EFFECTS OF ABUSE ON HEALTH

Several studies have found an additive effect of different types of childhood abuse experiences in predicting the severity of poor health outcomes (e.g., Arnow *et al.*, 2000; Diaz *et al.*, 2000; Felitti *et al.*, 1998; Golding *et al.*, 1997; Kessler 2000; Kessler *et al.*, 1997). For example, researchers found an additive effect of childhood sexual, physical, and emotional abuse on the number of distressing physical symptoms experienced (Walker *et al.*, 1999). In a large representative sample of women, those who experienced both childhood physical and sexual abuse were at increased risk of health problems in adulthood compared with women who experienced only one type of abuse (Thompson *et al.*, 2002). Felitti *et al.* (1998) found a relationship between the number of childhood abuse experiences (e.g., psychological, physical, emotional, and household dysfunction) and the occurrence of several specific medical problems (e.g., heart disease, cancer, chronic lung disease, skeletal fractures, and liver disease). However, in our research using the NCS data (Sachs-Ericsson *et al.*, 2005) contrary to expectations, individuals who experienced a combination of sexual and physical abuse did not have a higher frequency of health problems than those who experienced either type of abuse alone.

Nonetheless, understanding the independent implications of childhood sexual abuse and childhood physical abuse for health problems is important and can be complex because they often occur together, as well as with other negative childhood events (Felitti *et al.*, 1998; Kessler *et al.*, 1997; Mullen *et al.*, 1993; Romans *et al.*, 2002; Zuravin and Fontanella, 1999). For example, Felitti and colleagues (1998) found that when respondents experienced one childhood adversity, the probability of having experienced another was approximately 80 percent. Kessler (2000) argued that researchers often look at one childhood adversity, such as physical abuse, and assume subsequent problems are related to that, ignoring the possibility that physical abuse often occurs within a cluster of other childhood difficulties that may themselves account for the subsequent problems.

Similarly, Mullen and colleagues (Mullen *et al.*, 1993) argued that childhood abuse may be just one of several adverse experiences that occur within a context of family problems, and these other experiences may account for the relationship between abuse and negative life outcomes.

Researchers have documented that family characteristics associated with childhood abuse that contribute to the development of subsequent health-related problems may include parental psychopathology, family conflict, low socioeconomic status, parental loss or absence, and parental divorce (Felitti *et al.*, 1998; Fleming *et al.*, 1997; Kenny and McEachern, 2000; Molnar *et al.*, 2001; Romans *et al.*, 1995; Sidebotham and Golding, 2001; Zuravin and Fontanella, 1999). In order to understand the implications of each type of specific childhood adversity for health, it is important for researchers to try to distinguish their influence from other co-occurring childhood adversities.

In our work with the NCS sample, we have found that several family-of-origin variables were clearly associated with adult health problems (Sachs-Ericsson *et al.*, 2005). Specifically, parents' psychiatric disorders, parental abandonment, parental divorce, low levels of parental education, and family conflict were all associated with subsequent health problems. However, even after controlling for these family-of-origin factors, there remained a significant relationship between childhood abuse and health status (e.g., increased health problems and pain reports). Thus, our work supports the conclusion that both childhood sexual abuse and childhood physical abuse have an effect on subsequent health problems and pain reports independent of family-of-origin factors.

WHY DOES CHILDHOOD ABUSE AFFECT HEALTH FUNCTIONING?

Early abuse experiences may have an impact on adult health outcomes via several pathways. The physical and sexual abuse itself may cause physical damage resulting in subsequent health problems (Leserman et al., 1997). Sexual abuse may also result in sexually transmitted diseases (Hillis et al., 2000) or unwanted pregnancy (Dietz et al., 1999), and such problems may lead to subsequent health problems in adulthood. Further, individuals exposed to childhood abuse, as well as other childhood adversities, have been found to exhibit risky behaviors that can negatively influence health (Kendall-Tackett, 2002). These behaviors include increased use of alcohol and other drugs, driving while intoxicated, early onset of smoking, risky sexual behavior including multiple sex partners, decreased physical activity, compulsive eating and severe obesity (Felitti et al., 1998; Fleming et al., 1999; Kaplan et al., 1998; Nichols and Harlow, 2004; Springs and Friedrich, 1992; Walker et al., 1999; Williamson et al., 2002). Several of these behaviors and problems are associated with the leading causes of morbidity and mortality in the United States (Anderson et al., 1997).

Moreover, researchers have speculated that childhood abuse may increase the risk of health problems through comorbid psychiatric disorders. Further, a body of research has investigated the impact of early abuse experiences on the developing brain that has been found to influence immune functioning and sensitivity to stress, which may in turn contribute to increased health problems.

DO PSYCHIATRIC PROBLEMS INFLUENCE THE RELATIONSHIP BETWEEN CHILDHOOD ABUSE AND HEALTH PROBLEMS?

Researchers have postulated that psychiatric problems may mediate the influence of childhood abuse on health problems (Golding, 1994). Psychiatric problems are consistently found to be higher among individuals who have experienced childhood abuse (e.g., Kendler et al., 2000) and have been found to be related to health status (e.g., Schnurr and Spiro, 1999). Researchers have speculated that psychiatric disorders and the problems associated with such disorders, in turn, lead to higher rates of health problems. That is, childhood abuse may not be directly related to health problems but rather may have an indirect effect through the increased risk for psychiatric problems (Golding, 1994).

Studies have shown some support for the theory that psychiatric symptoms mediate the relationship between child abuse and adult health problems (Golding, 1999; Sachs-Ericsson *et al.*, 2005). However, the influence has been shown to be relatively minimal. For example, in their meta-analysis, Golding and colleagues (Golding *et al.*, 1997) concluded that depression did not markedly change the influence of abuse on subjective health.

In our research with the NCS sample, we found that lifetime psychiatric problems partially mediated the relationship between abuse and the occurrence of the one-year prevalence of serious health problems. That is, we found that childhood abuse was associated with an increase in lifetime psychiatric disorders, and increased psychiatric disorders were associated with increased health problems. When psychiatric problems were included in the analyses, the relationship between abuse and health problems decreased but still remained significant. Although the influence of psychiatric problems on the relationship between childhood abuse and health outcomes was significant, we concluded that its effects were relatively minimal. Nonetheless, our work with the NCS data, as well as other research, has shown that psychiatric disorders contribute to the relationship between abuse and health.

WHY MAY PSYCHIATRIC PROBLEMS INFLUENCE THE RELATIONSHIP BETWEEN ABUSE AND HEALTH?

How is it that psychiatric problems influence the relationship between abuse and health? Some of the same underlying processes that lead to an increase in vulnerability to psychiatric disorders among individuals who have experienced childhood abuse may lead to increased health problems (Kendall-Tackett, 2002). Such problems may include low self-esteem, poor coping skills, disturbed self-identity, poor interpersonal skills, insecure attachment styles, and increased vulnerability to stress (Becker-

Lausen and Mallon-Kraft, 1997; Romans *et al.*, 2002; Waldinger *et al.*, 2006). Further, individuals with a history of sexual assault were found to have less contact and received less support from friends and family (Golding *et al.*, 2002). Social support, in turn, has been repeatedly shown to be a major protective factor against psychiatric disorders, depression in particular (Plant and Sachs-Ericsson, 2004), and has also been shown to influence health outcomes (Israel *et al.*, 2002; Lett *et al.*, 2005).

CHILDHOOD ABUSE AND THE BRAIN: IMPLICATIONS FOR IMMUNE FUNCTIONING AND REACTIVITY TO STRESS

Early abuse experiences have been shown to affect the development of the brain (Heim and Nemeroff, 2002; Kendall-Tackett, 2002), which may contribute to suppressed immune functioning and increased physiological reactivity to stress, which, in turn, may increase vulnerability to health and psychiatric disorders. Specifically, abuse may cause chronic hyperarousal that may lead individuals to be more vulnerable to stress (Kendall-Tackett, 2002). Vulnerability to stress may be a diathesis for both psychiatric and health problems. For example, individuals with posttraumatic stress disorder (PTSD) and women who experienced childhood sexual abuse have been found to have enhanced sensitivity of the hypothalamic–pituitary–adrenal axis (Stein *et al.*, 1997; Yehuda *et al.*, 1995). Increased activity within this axis has been shown to suppress immune functioning (Altemus *et al.*, 2003).

Clinical evidence indicates that childhood abuse may increase the impact of negative life events on individuals' health by heightening their response to current stress. Thakkar and McCanne (2000) found that women with a history of abuse reported more physical symptoms in response to compounded daily stress than women with no abuse history. Researchers have demonstrated that the interaction between childhood abuse and adulthood stress is a strong predictor of adrenocorticotropin responsiveness to psychosocial stressors. This responsiveness, in turn, may influence physical health by suppressing immune functioning (Altemus *et al.*, 2003; Heim and Nemeroff, 2002). Parallel to these investigations are studies of general (non-abused) populations, which have found that an increase in daily stress is associated with a decline in general health (DeLongis *et al.*, 1988; Evans and Edgerton, 1991; Stone *et al.*, 1987). Based on these converging findings, it appears that current stressful life events may influence the relationship between childhood abuse and adult health problems.

In our work with the NCS data, we indeed found that current stressful life events moderated the relationship between childhood abuse and adult health problems. Specifically, the presence of stress more than doubled the effect of any abuse (physical or sexual) on health problems. In other words, current life stressors substantially contribute to poor health for those who have been abused (Cromer and Sachs-Ericsson, 2006). Our findings are consistent with past research on the relationship between childhood abuse and the sensitization of stress-responsive neurobiological systems, as well as the dysregulation of the immune system. Specifically, Heim and colleagues (Heim *et al.*, 2002) have suggested that childhood abuse is associated with increased neuroendocrine stress reactivity. This reactivity is further increased in the presence of trauma in adulthood. A separate line of research has suggested that life stressors and childhood abuse are associated with a weakening of the immune system (Golding, 1994; Kimerling and Calhoun, 1994; Pennebaker and Susman, 1988), which could increase an individual's vulnerability to disease when exposed to subsequent stressors (Koss *et al.*, 1990).

It is also possible that there may be a hyperactivation of the immune system present in individuals who have experienced childhood abuse. Dysregulation of the immune system may also be related to the increase in psychiatric comorbidity among individuals with abuse histories. Specifically, individuals with PTSD (resulting from childhood sexual abuse) display several markers of increased immune activation (Wilson *et al.*, 1999). Moreover, depression, which is highly comorbid with childhood abuse, has also been associated with impaired immune functioning, with increased cytokine secretion and dysregulation of cortisol implicated as mechanisms by which the immune system may be suppressed (Connor and Leonard, 1998; Maes *et al.*, 1995).

This paradigm of immune dysregulation among individuals with childhood abuse is consistent with NCS data, which indicates that autoimmune problems are more frequent in individuals with a history of childhood abuse. Thus, it seems that immunological research, in conjunction with research on childhood abuse, is a promising area for future investigations.

WHY IS CHILDHOOD ABUSE RELATED TO PAIN?

Several theories have been put forth to account for the association between painful medical conditions and childhood abuse. Kendall-Tackett (2001) suggested that childhood abuse may contribute to a negative attributional style (Sachs-Ericsson *et al.*, 2006) an inability to manage stress (Kendall-Tackett, 2001), and limited social support (Golding *et al.*, 2002), each of which may exacerbate pain. Furthermore, according to the gate-control theory (Melzack and Wall, 1965), cognitions, beliefs, and emotion influence pain perception. That is, there are psychological and physical factors that influence the brain's interpretation of painful sensations. Researchers have suggested that trauma-related alterations in neurosensory processing may amplify pain (Arnow *et al.*, 2000), and childhood abuse may lower thresholds for labeling painful stimuli as noxious (Scarinci *et al.*, 1994).

Interestingly, in a recent experimental study, findings suggest that individuals with a history of childhood abuse may have a "decreased sensitivity" to experimentally induced pain; however, they may have more chronic pain-related difficulties. As the authors note, their research highlights the complexity of the relationship between abuse history and pain, thereby illustrating the need for further investigation of pain-related correlates of abuse (Fillingim and Edwards, 2005).

WHY MAY DEPRESSION INFLUENCE THE RELATIONSHIP BETWEEN CHILDHOOD ABUSE AND PAIN?

Researchers have suggested that the increased pain reports associated with individuals who have been abused may be related to increased psychiatric comorbidity and, in particular, depression. Depression is common among adult survivors of abuse (Goldberg, 1994; Levitan *et al.*, 1998; Molnar *et al.*, 2001; Roosa *et al.*, 1999; Turner and Muller, 2004; Zuravin and Fontanella, 1999), as well as among chronic pain patients (Faucett, 1994; Fishbain *et al.*, 1997; Magni *et al.*, 1994; McWilliams *et al.*, 2003). Moreover, past research has shown that depression increases pain reports among individuals with health problems (Hernandez and Sachs-Ericsson, 2006).

Biologically, the related neurochemistry underlying both depression and pain may enhance their association. Specifically, depression is associated with a neurochemical imbalance of neurotransmitters (Bair *et al.*, 2003; Fava, 2003), including serotonin, norepinephrine, and dopamine (Andrews and Pinder, 2000; Blackburn-Munro and Blackburn-Munro, 2001). Analgesic effects are produced by serotonin and norepinephrine through descending pain pathways, and these effects may be disrupted by decreased levels of these neurotransmitters (Andrews and Pinder, 2000; Blackburn-Munro and Blackburn-Munro, 2001). The pain modulation system influences affect and attention to peripheral stimuli and plays a role in suppressing minor signals coming from the body (Blackburn-Munro and Blackburn-Munro, 2001; Stahl, 2002). These signals may be less suppressed when serotonin and norepinephrine are depleted (Bair *et al.*, 2003). Thus, the association between pain and depression may be due, in part, to the neurochemical impact depression plays in the pain response (Blackburn-Munro and Blackburn-Munro, 2001).

Emotionally negative mood states may also reduce tolerance to aversive stimuli (Meagher *et al.*, 2001; Zelman *et al.*, 1991). The motivational priming model proposes that negative emotional states enhance pain perception while pleasant affective states attenuate it. Specifically, studies have shown that negative affective states decreased pain tolerance to aversive stimuli while positive affective states increased tolerance to aversive stimuli (Meagher *et al.*, 2001; Zelman *et al.*, 1991). Thus, negative affective states of depressed individuals may magnify their experience of pain.

In our research using the NCS data, we found that participants who experienced childhood abuse reported more pain in relation to their health problems compared to those participants without abuse histories. We had also hypothesized that because childhood abuse is associated with higher rates of depression and depression is associated with more reported pain, depression would mediate the relationship between childhood abuse and adult pain reports. Indeed, we did find higher rates of pain reports, as well as higher rates of depression, among abuse survivors. Whereas we found initially that depression mediated the relationship between childhood abuse and pain reports, after controlling for differences between the abused and non-abused participants on specific health problems (which were greater among the abused participants), depression was not found to mediate the relationship. Thus, we concluded that the higher rate of depression found among adults who experienced childhood abuse was not the primary factor for their increased pain reports. Rather, childhood abuse and depression contributed independently to pain reports (Sachs-Ericsson *et al.*, 2007). Thus, both depression and pain, common sequelae of childhood abuse, need to be appropriately addressed within the context of medical and psychological treatments.

TREATMENT IMPLICATIONS

This chapter has highlighted the connection between abuse history and poor adult health functioning. Considering the costs, both personal and societal, that are associated with this relationship, continued research on etiological mechanisms and the development of abuse-preventive measures is vital. Of more immediate and practical importance is a number of treatment implications and recommendations that arise from the association between abuse, medical problems, and mental health functioning (Schnurr and Green, 2004).

IDENTIFYING PATIENTS WITH A HISTORY OF CHILDHOOD ABUSE
The first step necessary in attenuating the psychological and physical health consequences of trauma is to identify those individuals presenting for medical care or mental health treatment who have experienced childhood abuse (Schnurr and Green, 2004). From a holistic perspective, the accurate diagnosis of both physical and mental illnesses is a key step in improving a patient's overall health. Mental health professionals need to consider the patient's physical as well as his or her mental health in the context of an overall treatment plan. Moreover, from a primary care standpoint, knowledge of trauma history and the state of a patient's mental health can aid in developing the most appropriate and effective treatment plan (Schnurr and Green, 2004). This emphasizes the need for practitioners to identify individuals with past abuse history and to screen for health problems as well as for psychiatric disorders.

INITIAL SCREENING
For a typical medical setting, the most cost-effective method to identify psychiatric symptoms would be to employ a variety of initial screening methods, in combination with referrals to appropriate agencies (Green and Kimmerling, 2004). Schoenbaum and colleagues (Schoenbaum et al., 2001) have discussed the success of using universal screening procedures with regard to depression, and it is possible that similar methods could aid in the identification of other psychiatric disorders that are commonly associated with childhood abuse, such as PTSD and other anxiety disorders. We also would hope that both medical and mental health practitioners who work with adult survivors of childhood abuse will assess their clients for chronic pain and make referrals as necessary. Chronic pain can impact both their clients' physical and emotional well-being, and any

treatment that ignores it will be incomplete. Screening for pain can initially be completed with the use of a one- or two-item pain measure. Pain is a subjective experience that is assessed predominately through the individual's subjective self-report (e.g., Please rate your current experience of pain on a scale from 0 to 10, with 0 being "No pain", and 10 being "Intense Pain"). Researchers have used these single-item self-report measures of pain, and research supports the validity of such measures.

It will also be advisable for mental health professionals to identify those individuals within their care who may be at risk for serious health problems. One helpful step may be for clinicians to assess patients' general physical health history in conjunction with their mental health history. Furthermore, mental health practitioners may wish to refer their patients to a non-psychiatric physician to aid in the detection of any potential medical problems (DeVellis and DeVellis, 2001). It is important that individuals' medical problems be appropriately addressed, and psychotherapy treatments should specifically address psychological and behavioral variables that may contribute to or exacerbate the medically related conditions (e.g., risky health behaviors, catastrophizing cognitions related to physical symptoms). Clinicians should inform and educate their patients on the association between physical health, pain, and psychological distress. Raising awareness in this way will lead to greater focus on the physical manifestation of mental illness, which can in turn aid in the individual obtaining appropriate treatment for both physical and mental health functioning.

IMPLICATIONS FOR HEALTH CARE PRACTICE

The connection between abuse history and mental and physical health has a number of general implications for health care practice, which may enhance the delivery of care to survivors of childhood abuse (Monahan and Forgash, 2000; Schachter et al., 2004). These include increasing a patient's sense of safety, approaching the disclosure of childhood abuse in an open and empathic manner, and being sensitive to abuse-related issues (e.g., boundaries, effects of trauma on the body, potential for flashback triggers). Consistent with the principles of self-determination theory (Sheldon *et al.*, 2003), Schachter and colleagues (Schachter *et al.*, 2004) found that a general approach is to treat the clinician–patient relationship as a type of collaborative partnership. This approach encourages the patient to be more in control of deciding a treatment course. Further, by educating individuals on their illness and available treatment options, abuse survivors will feel more respected and are more likely to have greater treatment adherence.

MONITOR FOR HIGH-RISK BEHAVIORS
In addition to the more general implications discussed above, there are several specific treatment guidelines and recommendations. These include the monitoring of health risk behaviors, the reduction of current life stress, and efforts to strengthen social support. Research has established a number of health behaviors and lifestyle factors (e.g., smoking and substance use) as the leading causes of morbidity and mortality in the U.S. (Kendall-Tackett, 2001), and these health-risk behaviors often represent the most proximal causes of disease or death. Researchers have furthermore shown that adverse childhood experiences contribute to the development of these harmful health behaviors and lifestyle factors (e.g., substance use, driving while intoxicated, obesity, risky sexual experiences, and early onset of smoking (Kaplan *et al.*, 1998; Springs and Friedrich, 1992; Walker *et al.*, 1999; Williamson *et al.*, 2002)). With regard to treatment, it will be important for primary care physicians to screen and monitor these behaviors, given their connection to many medical problems. From a mental health perspective, it will also be efficacious to screen and monitor these behaviors as they may represent poor coping skills used to deal with trauma-associated psychological distress (e.g., Springs and Friedrich, 1992). Importantly, these coping skills can be replaced during therapy with healthier strategies from both a mental and physical health standpoint.

REDUCE CURRENT LIFE STRESS

A second specific treatment recommendation is the reduction of current life stress. As outlined in this chapter, a growing body of literature indicates that current life stress can exacerbate the relationship between trauma and poor health (e.g., Cromer and Sachs-Ericsson, 2006; Evans and Edgerton, 1991). Moreover, stress is an important factor in the onset and relapse of most psychiatric disorders (Rende and Plomin, 1992). Education on this relationship can empower patients, and a component of treatment can be aimed at methods for reducing psychosocial stressors.

STRENGTHEN SOCIAL SUPPORT NETWORKS

A third specific recommendation is the strengthening of social support networks. Biggs and colleagues (Biggs *et al.*, 2004) have found the greatest impairment in health functioning among individuals with a history of childhood abuse who also have a disparity in social support. Similarly, Kimerling and Calhoun (1994) found that supportive responses to disclosures of assault may act as a buffer against increased health problems. Further, social support has been shown to be an important buffer against psychiatric disorders, and in particular depression (Petty *et al.*, 2004). Thus, one aspect of psychological interventions may be to incorporate a component that enhances a supportive environment for individuals with an abuse history.

There are several psychotherapy protocols that focus on increasing interpersonal skills and reducing reactivity to stress. For example, dialectical behavior therapy has a focus in building interpersonal relationships, increasing stress tolerance, and developing self-soothing behaviors (Comtois and Linehan, 2006). Exposure-based therapies (proven to be efficacious for several anxiety disorders) appear to be helpful for individuals with an abuse history who have health-related problems (Leserman, 2005). However, as Leserman (2005) notes, we need more research examining psychological treatments that might be efficacious in treating the physical health problems associated with sexual abuse history.

CARE FOR PATIENTS WITH CHRONIC PAIN

In treating individuals with chronic pain, our research suggests that childhood abuse and depression contribute independently to pain experiences. For those individuals who have experienced childhood abuse and have comorbid pain and depression, addressing one problem without the other would likely be insufficient in adequately meeting their treatment needs. Many of the same recommendations described above for increasing social skills, increasing social support networks and decreasing stress are also applicable to the treatments of comorbid pain and depression among individuals with a history of abuse. In addition, both depression and chronic pain can be treated with antidepressants, which will help alleviate both their pain and depression. Further, these health- and pain-related problems can be treated with exercise, physical and occupational therapy, stress management, and activity pacing. Patients' catastrophizing beliefs about their health can also be addressed with the use of cognitive behavioral psychotherapy. All of these approaches have been found to be helpful in reducing chronic pain (Kendall-Tackett *et al.*, 2003).

As Schnurr and Green (2004) and others have noted, the association between trauma, mental health, and medical problems has "systems" and policy implications. The above recommendations, when taken altogether, may seem daunting given our current health care system. However, there exists the need for primary care practitioners and mental health clinicians to collaborate on the delivery of the most effective care for individuals with abuse histories. An integrated care model can more effectively accomplish the preceding treatment recommendations. Although more research needs to be conducted on the integration of physical and mental health treatment, initial studies indicate that the simultaneous treatment of psychological disorders can substantially reduce health care utilization, dramatically increase treatment adherence, and lead to better recovery (e.g., Kimerling and Calhoun, 1994). Until better abuse-preventative measures are developed, both the medical and psychiatric community should attempt to integrate these recommendations into their practice, potentially exploring more robust collaborations with one another. In so doing, they will be able to provide abuse survivors with the most effective and holistic treatment of the psychological and physical sequalae of trauma exposure.

CONCLUSIONS AND FUTURE RESEARCH

Future epidemiological studies that assess childhood abuse early in an individual's life, and then tracks the onset and course of subsequent health problems, would contribute greatly to our understanding of the relationship between abuse and adult health problems. Our research, based on a large representative epidemiological sample, has extended past research by demonstrating a relationship between childhood sexual and physical abuse and increased rates of overall health problems, and the subsequent occurrence of several specific health problems. Moreover, we found that among participants with abuse histories, health problems were associated with increased report of pain. Further, our work has shown that current life stressors moderate the relationship between abuse and health problems such that, in the presence of stress, health problems are greater among those with abuse histories.

Whereas several researchers have speculated that increased rates of health problems and higher pain reports among individuals with abuse histories may be related to an increase in psychiatric comorbidity, our work and the work of others has shown that psychiatric disorders have a relatively minor influence on the relationship of abuse, health problems, and pain reports. From our data it appears that health problems, chronic pain, and psychiatric disorders are all sequelae of past abuse. That conclusion should change the way we approach treatment of patients. Each of these problems needs to be addressed in treatment. Addressing one problem and not the other would likely be insufficient in adequately meeting the individual's treatment needs.

The continuing influence of childhood abuse on adult health functioning, as well as the impact of current stress, underscores the significant public health concern surrounding childhood abuse. Various mechanisms most likely underlie the association between childhood abuse and poor health, some of which we have reviewed in the current chapter. Future research identifying and elaborating upon these underlying mechanisms will play an important role in extending our understanding of the negative sequalae of childhood abuse.

REFERENCES

Altemus, M., Cloitre, M., and Dhabhar, F.S. (2003). Enhanced cellular immune response in women with PTSD related to childhood abuse. *American Journal of Psychiatry, 160*, 1705–1707.

Anderson R.N., Kochanek, K.D., and Murphy. S.L. (1997). *Report of final mortality statistics, 1995*. Monthly vital statistics report, *45*(11), supp 2. Hyattsville, MD: National Center for Health Statistics.

Andrews, J., and Pinder, R. (2000). Antidepressants of the future: A critical assessment of the chemistry and pharmacology of novel antidepressants in development. In M.J. Parnham and B.J. Parnham (eds), *Antidepressants: Milestones in drug therapy* (pp. 115–157). Boston, MA: Birkhauser.

Arnow, B., Hart, S., Hayward, C., Dea, R., and Barr Taylor, C. (2000). Severity of child maltreatment, pain complaints and medical utilization among women. *Journal of Psychiatric Research, 34*(6), 413–421.

Bair, M.J., Robinson, R.L., Katon, W., and Kroenke, K. (2003). Depression and pain comorbidity: A literature review. *Archives of Internal Medicine, 163*(20), 2433–2445.

Becker-Lausen, E., and Mallon-Kraft, S. (1997). Pandemic outcomes: The intimacy variable. In G.K. Kantor and J.S. Jasinski (eds), *Out of darkness: Current perspectives on family violence* (pp. 49–57). Newbury Park, CA: Sage.

Bendixen, M., Muus, K., and Schei, B. (1994). The impact of child sexual abuse – A study of a random sample of Norwegian students. *Child Abuse and Neglect, 18*(10), 837–847.

Biggs, A-M., Aziz, Q., Tomenson, B., and Creed, F. (2003). Do childhood adversity and recent social stress predict health care use in patients presenting with upper abdominal or chest pain? *Psychosomatic Medicine, 65*(6), 1020–1028.

Biggs, A-M., Aziz, Q., Tomenson, B., and Creed, F. (2004). Effect of childhood adversity on health related quality of life in patients with upper abdominal or chest pain. *Gut, 53*(2), 180–186.

Blackburn-Munro, G., and Blackburn-Munro, R. (2001). Chronic pain, chronic stress and depression: Coincidence or consequence? *Journal of Neuroendocrinology, 13*(12), 1009–1023.

Boisset-Pioro, M., Esdaile, J., and Fitzcharles, M. (1995). Sexual and physical abuse in women with fibromyalgia syndrome. *Arthritis and Rheumatism, 38*(2), 235–241.

Comtois, K., and Linehan, M. (2006). Psychosocial treatments of suicidal behaviors: A practice-friendly review. *Journal of Clinical Psychology, 62*(2), 161–170.

Connor, T.J., and Leonard, B.E. (1998). Depression, stress and immunological activation: The role of cytokines in depressive disorders. *Life Sciences, 62*, 583–606.

Cromer, K., and Sachs-Ericsson, N. (2006). The association between childhood abuse and the occurrence of adult health problems: Moderation via current life stress. *Journal of Traumatic Stress, 6*, 967–971.

DeLongis, A., Folkman, S., and Lazarus, R. (1988). The impact of daily stress on health and mood: Psychological and social resources as mediators. *Journal of Personality and Social Psychology, 54*(3), 486–495.

DeVellis, B.M., and DeVellis, R.F. (2001). Self-efficacy and health. In A. Baum, T.A. Evenson and J.E. Singer (eds), *Handbook of health psychology* (pp. 235–248). Mahwaw, NJ: Erlbaum.

Diaz, A., Simantov, E., and Rickert, V.I. (2000). Effect of abuse on health: Results of a national survey. *Archives of Pediatric Adolescent Medicine, 156*, 811–817.

Dietz, P.M., Spitz, A.M., Anda, R.F., Williamson, D.F., McMahon, P.M., Santelli, J.S., *et al.* (1999). Unintended pregnancy among adult women exposed to abuse or household dysfunction during their childhood. *Journal of the American Medical Association, 282*, 1359–1364.

Dong, M., Giles, W.H., Felitti, V.J., Dube, S.R., Williams, J.E., Chapman, D.P., *et al.* (2004). Insights into causal pathways for ischemic heart disease: Adverse Childhood Experiences Study. *Circulation, 110*(13), 1761–1766.

Drossman, D.A. (1994). Physical and sexual abuse and gastrointestinal illness: What is the link? *American Journal of Medicine, 97*(2), 105–107.

Drossman, D.A., Talley, N.J., Leserman, J., Olden, K.W., and Barreiro, M.A. (1995). Sexual and physical abuse and gastrointestinal illness: Review and recommendations. *Annals of Internal Medicine, 123*, 782–794.

Drossman, D.A., Leserman, J., Li, Z., Keefe, F., Hu, Y.J.B., and Toomey, T.C. (2000). Effects of coping on health outcome among women with gastrointestinal disorders. *Psychosomatic Medicine, 62*(3), 309–317.

Evans, P.D., and Edgerton, N. (1991). Life-events and mood as predictors of the common cold. *British Journal of Medical Psychology, 64*(1), 35–44.

Faucett, J. (1994). Depression in painful chronic disorders: The role of pain and conflict about pain. *Journal of Pain Symptom Management, 9*(8), 520–526.

Fava, M. (2003). The role of the serotonergic and noradrenergic neurotransmitter systems in the treatment of psychological and physical symptoms of depression. *Journal of Clinical Psychiatry, 64 Suppl 13*, 26–29.

Felitti, V.J., Anda, R.F., Nordenberg, D., Williamson, D.F., Spitz, A.M., Edwards, V., *et al.* (1998). Relationship of childhood abuse and household dysfunction to many of the leading causes of death in adults. The Adverse Childhood Experiences (ACE) Study. *American Journal of Preventative Medicine, 14*, 245–258.

Fillingim, R., and Edwards, R. (2005). Is self-reported childhood abuse history associated with pain perception among healthy young women and men? *Clinical Journal of Pain, 21*(5), 387–397.

Finestone, H., Stenn, P., Davies, F., Stalker, C., Fry, R., and Koumanis, J. (2000). Chronic pain and health care utilization in women with a history of childhood sexual abuse. *Child Abuse and Neglect, 24*(4), 547–556.

Fishbain, D., Cutler, R., Rosomoff, H., and Rosomoff, R. (1997). Chronic pain-associated depression: Antecedent or consequence of chronic pain? A review. *Clinical Journal of Pain, 13*(2), 116–137.

Fleming, J., Mullen, P., and Bammer, G. (1997). A study of potential risk factors for sexual abuse in childhood. *Child Abuse and Neglect, 21*(1), 49–58.

Fleming, J., Mullen, P.E., Sibthorpe, B., and Bammer, G. (1999). The long-term impact of childhood sexual abuse in Australian women. *Child Abuse and Neglect, 23*(2), 145–159.

Goldberg, R. (1994). Childhood abuse, depression, and chronic pain. *Clinical Journal of Pain, 10*(4), 277–281.

Golding, J.M. (1994). Sexual assault history and physical health in randomly selected Los Angeles women. *Health Psychology, 13*, 130–138.

Golding, J.M. (1999). Sexual-assault history and long-term physical health problems: Evidence from clinical and population epidemiology. *Current Directions in Psychological Science, 8*(6), 191–194.

Golding, J.M., Cooper, M.L., and George, L.K. (1997). Sexual assault history and health perceptions: Seven general population studies. *Health Psychology, 16*, 417–425.

Golding, J.M., Wilsnack, S.C., and Cooper, M. (2002). Sexual assault history and social support: Six general population studies. *Journal of Traumatic Stress, 15*(3), 187–197.

Golding, J.M., Wilsnack, S.C., and Learman, L.A. (1998). Prevalence of sexual assault history among women with common gynecologic symptoms. *American Journal of Obstetrics and Gynecology, 179*, 1013–1019.

Goodwin, R.D., Hoven, C.W., Murison, R., and Hotopf, M. (2003). Association between childhood physical abuse and gastrointestinal disorders and migraine in adulthood. *American Journal of Public Health, 93*(7), 1065–1067.

Green, B.L., and Kimmerling, R. (2004). Trauma, posttraumatic stress disorder, and health status. In P. Schnurr and B.L. Green (eds), *Trauma and health: Physical health consequences of exposure in extreme stress* (pp. 129–155). Washington, DC: American Psychological Association.

Green, C., Flowe-Valencia, H., Rosenblum, L., and Tait, A. (2001). The role of childhood and adulthood abuse among women presenting for chronic pain management. *Clinical Journal of Pain, 17*(4), 359–364.

Harlow, B.L., and Stewart, E.G. (2005). Adult-onset vulvodynia in relation to childhood violence victimization. *American Journal of Epidemiology, 161*(9), 871–880.

Heim, C., and Nemeroff, C.B. (2002). Neurobiology of early life stress: Clinical studies. *Seminar in Clinical Neuropsychiatry, 7*, 147–159.

Heim, C., Newport, D.J., Wagner, D., Wilcox, M.M., Miller, A.H., and Nemeroff, C.B. (2002). The role of early adverse experience and adulthood stress in the prediction of neuroendocrine stress reactivity in women: A multiple regression analysis. *Depression and Anxiety, 15*(3), 117–125.

Hernandez, A., and Sachs-Ericsson, N. (2006). Ethnic differences in pain reports and the moderating role of depression in a community sample of Hispanic and Caucasian participants with serious health problems. *Psychosomatic Medicine, 68*(1), 121–128.

Hillis, S.D., Anda, R.F., Felitti, V.J., Nordenberg, D., and Marchbanks, P.A. (2000). Adverse childhood experiences and sexually transmitted diseases in men and women: A retrospective study. *Pediatrics, 106*, 11.

Israel, B.A., Farquhar, S.A., Schulz, A.J., James, S.A., and Parker, E.A. (2002). The relationship between social support, stress, and health among women on Detroit's east side. *Health Education and Behavior, 29*(3), 342–360.

Jamieson, D., and Steege, J. (1997). The association of sexual abuse with pelvic pain complaints in a primary care population. *American Journal of Obstetrics and Gynecology, 177*(6), 1408–1412.

Kaplan, S.J., Pelcovitz, D., Salzinger, S., Weiner, M., Mandel, F.S., and Lesser, M.L. (1998). Adolescent physical abuse: Risk for adolescent psychiatric disorders. *American Journal of Psychiatry, 155*(7), 954–959.

Kendall-Tackett, K.A. (2001). Chronic pain: The next frontier in child maltreatment research. *Child Abuse and Neglect, 25*(8), 997–1000.

Kendall-Tackett, K.A. (2002). The health effects of childhood abuse: Four pathways by which abuse can influence health. *Child Abuse and Neglect, 26*, 715–729.

Kendall-Tackett, K.A., and Marshall, R. (1999). Victimization and diabetes: An exploratory study. *Child Abuse and Neglect, 23*, 593–596.

Kendall-Tackett, K.A., Marshall, R., and Ness, K.E. (2003). Chronic pain syndromes and violence against women. *Women and Therapy, 26*, 45–56.

Kendler, K.S., Bulik, C.M., Silberg, J., Hettema, J.M., Myers, J., and Prescott, C.A. (2000). Childhood sexual abuse and adult psychiatric and substance use disorders in women: An epidemiological and co-twin control analysis. *Archives of General Psychiatry, 57*, 953–959.

Kenny, M.C., and McEachern, A.G. (2000). Racial, ethnic, and cultural factors of childhood sexual abuse: A selected review of the literature. *Clinical Psychology Review, 20*, 905–922.

Kessler, R.C. (2000). The long-term effects of childhood adversities on depression and other psychiatric disorders. In T. O. Harris (ed.), *Where inner and outer worlds meet* (pp. 227–244). London: Routledge

Kessler, R.C., Davis, C.G., and Kendler, K.S. (1997). Childhood adversity and adult psychiatric disorder in the US National Comorbidity Survey. *Psychological Medicine, 27*, 1101–1119.

Kimerling, R., and Calhoun, K.S. (1994). Somatic symptoms, social support, and treatment seeking among sexual assault victims. *Journal of Consulting and Clinical Psychology, 62*(2), 333–340.

Kopec, J., and Sayre, E. (2004). Traumatic experiences in childhood and the risk of arthritis: A prospective cohort study. *Canadian Journal of Public Health, 95*(5), 361–365.

Koss, M.P., Woodruff, W.J., and Koss, P.G. (1990). Relation of criminal victimization to health perceptions among women medical patients. *Journal of Consulting and Clinical Psychology, 58*(2), 147–152.

Lampe, A., Doering, S., Rumpold, G., Soelder, E., Krismer, M., Kantner-Rumplmair, W., *et al.* (2003). Chronic pain syndromes and their relation to childhood abuse and stressful life events. *Journal of Psychosomatic Research, 54*, 361–367.

Latthe, P., Mignini, L., Gray, R., Hills, R., and Khan, K. (2006). Factors predisposing women to chronic pelvic pain: Systematic review. *British Medical Journal, 332*(7544), 749–755.

Leserman, J. (2005). Sexual abuse history: Prevalence, health effects, mediators, and psychological treatment. *Psychosomatic Medicine, 67*(6), 906–915.

Leserman, J., Drossman, D.A., Li, Z., Toomey, T.C., Nachman, G., and Glogau, L. (1996). Sexual and physical abuse history in gastroenterology practice: How types of abuse impact health status. *Psychosomatic Medicine, 58*(1), 4–15.

Leserman, J., Li, Z., Drossman, D.A., Toomey, T.C., Nachman, G., and Glogau, L. (1997). Impact of sexual and physical abuse dimensions on health status: Development of an abuse severity measure. *Psychosomatic Medicine, 59*, 152–160.

Lett, H.S., Blumenthal, J.A., Babyak, M.A., Strauman, T.J., Robins, C., and Sherwood, A. (2005). Social support and coronary heart disease: Epidemiologic evidence and implications for treatment. *Psychosomatic Medicine, 67*(6), 869–878.

Levitan, R.D., Parikh, S.V., Lesage, A.D., Hegadoren, K.M., Adams, M., Kennedy, S.H., *et al.* (1998). Major depression in individuals with a history of childhood physical or sexual abuse: Relationship to neurovegetative features, mania, and gender. *American Journal of Psychiatry, 155*(12), 1746–1752.

Linton, S.J. (1997). A population-based study of the relationship between sexual abuse and back pain: Establishing a link. *Pain, 73*(1), 47–53.

Linton, S.J. (2002). A prospective study of the effects of sexual or physical abuse on back pain. *Pain, 96*(3), 347–351.

Maes, M., Bosmans, E., and Meltzer, H.Y. (1995). Immunoendocrine aspects of major depression. Relationships between plasma interleukin-6 and soluble interleukin-2 receptor, prolactin and cortisol. *European Archives of Psychiatry and Clinical Neuroscience, 245*, 172–178.

Magni, G., Moreschi, C., Rigatti-Luchini, S., and Merskey, H. (1994). Prospective study on the relationship between depressive symptoms and chronic musculoskeletal pain. *Pain, 56*(3), 289–297.

McBeth, J., Macfarlane, G., Benjamin, S., Morris, S., and Silman, A. (1999). The association between tender points, psychological distress, and adverse childhood experiences: A community-based study. *Arthritis and Rheumatism, 42*(7), 1397–1404.

McWilliams, L., Cox, B., and Enns, M. (2003). Mood and anxiety disorders associated with chronic pain: An examination in a nationally representative sample. *Pain, 106*(1–2), 127–133.

Meagher, M.W., Arnau, R.C., and Rhudy, J.L. (2001). Pain and emotion: Effects of affective picture modulation. *Psychosomatic Medicine, 63*(1), 79–90.

Melzack, R., and Wall, P. (1965). Pain mechanisms: A new theory. *Science, 150*, 171–179.

Molnar, B., Buka, S., and Kessler, R. (2001). Child sexual abuse and subsequent psychopathology: Results from the National Comorbidity Survey. *American Journal of Public Health, 91*(5), 753–760.

Monahan, K., and Forgash, C. (2000). Enhancing the health care experiences of adult female survivors of childhood sexual abuse. *Women Health, 30*(4), 27–41.

Mullen, P., Martin, J., Anderson, J., Romans, S., and Herbison, G. (1993). Childhood sexual abuse and mental health in adult life. *British Journal of Psychiatry, 163*(6), 721–732.

Newman, M., Clayton, L., Zuellig, A., Cashman, L., Arnow, B., Dea, R., *et al.* (2000). The relationship of childhood sexual abuse and depression with somatic symptoms and medical utilization. *Psychological Medicine, 30*(5), 1063–1077.

Nichols, H.B., and Harlow, B.L. (2004). Childhood abuse and risk of smoking onset. *Journal of Epidemiology and Community Health, 58*(5), 402–406.

Pennebaker, J.W., and Susman, J.R. (1988). Disclosure of traumas and psychosomatic processes. *Social Science and Medicine, 26*(3), 327–332.

Petty, C., Sachs-Ericsson, N., and Joiner, T. (2004). Interpersonal dysfunction: Cause or result of depressive disorders. *Journal of Affective Disorders, 81*(2), 115–122.

Plant, E.A., and Sachs-Ericsson, N. (2004). Racial and ethnic differences in depression: The roles of social support and meeting basic needs. *Journal of Consulting and Clinical Psychology, 72*(1), 41–52.

Raphael, K., Chandler, H., and Ciccone, D. (2004). Is childhood abuse a risk factor for chronic pain in adulthood? *Current Pain and Headache Report, 8*(2), 99–110.

Raphael, K., Widom, C., and Lange, G. (2001). Childhood victimization and pain in adulthood: A prospective investigation. *Pain, 92*(1–2), 283–293.

Rende, R., and Plomin, R. (1992). Diathesis-stress models of psychopathology: A quantitative genetic perspective. *Applied and Preventive Psychology, 1*(4), 177–182.

Romans, S., Belaise, C., Martin, J., Morris, E., and Raffi, A. (2002). Childhood abuse and later medical disorders in women. An epidemiological study. *Psychotherapy and Psychosomatics, 71*(3), 141–150.

Romans, S., Martin, J., Anderson, J., O'Shea, M., and Mullen, P. (1995). Factors that mediate between child sexual abuse and adult psychological outcome. *Psychological Medicine, 25*(1), 127–142.

Roosa, M., Reinholtz, C., and Angelini, P. (1999). The relation of child sexual abuse and depression in young women: Comparisons across four ethnic groups. *Journal of Abnormal Child Psychology, 27*(1), 65–76.

Sachs-Ericsson, N., Kendall-Tackett, K., and Hernandez, A. (2007). Childhood abuse, chronic pain and depression in the National Comorbidity Survey. *Child Abuse and Neglect, 31*(5), 531–547.

Sachs-Ericsson, N., Blazer, D., Plant, E.A., and Arnow, B. (2005). Childhood sexual and physical abuse and the one-year prevalence of medical problems in the National Comorbidity Study. *Health Psychology, 24*(1), 32–40.

Sachs-Ericsson, N., Verona, E., Joiner, T., and Preacher, K. (2006). Parental verbal abuse and the mediating role of self-criticism in adult internalizing disorders. *Journal of Affective Disorders, 93*(1–3), 71–78.

Scarinci, I.C., McDonald-Haile, J., Bradley, L.A., and Richter, J.E. (1994). Altered pain perception and psychosocial features among women with gastrointestinal disorders and history of abuse: A preliminary model. *The American Journal of Medicine, 97*(2), 108–118.

Schachter, C.L., Radomsky, N.A., Stalker, C.A., and Teram, E. (2004). Women survivors of child sexual abuse. How can health professionals promote healing? *Canadian Family Physician, 50*, 405–412.

Schnurr, P., and Green, B.L. (2004). Understanding relationships among trauma, post-traumatic stress disorder, and health outcomes. *Advances in Mind–Body Medicine, 20*(1), 18–29.

Schnurr, P.P., and Spiro, A. (1999). Combat exposure, posttraumatic stress disorder symptoms, and health behaviors as predictors of self-reported physical health in older veterans. *Journal of Nervous and Mental Disorders, 187*, 353–359.

Schoenbaum, M., Unutzer, J., Sherbourne, C., Duan, N., Rubenstein, L.V., Miranda, J., *et al.* (2001). Cost-effectiveness of practice-initiated quality improvement for depression: Results of a randomized controlled trial. *Journal of the American Medical Association, 286*(11), 1325–1330.

Sheldon, K., Williams, G., and Joiner, T. (2003). *Motivating physical and mental health: Applying self-determination theory in the clinic.* New Haven, CT: Yale University Press.

Sidebotham, P., and Golding, J. (2001). Child maltreatment in the "children of the nineties": A longitudinal study of parental risk factors. *Child Abuse and Neglect, 25*(9), 1177–1200.

Springs, F.E., and Friedrich, W.N. (1992). Health risk behaviors and medical sequelae of childhood sexual abuse. *Mayo Clinic Proceedings, 67*, 527–532.

Stahl, S. (2002). Does depression hurt? *Journal of Clinical Psychiatry, 63*(4), 273–274.

Stein, M.B., and Barrett-Connor, E. (2000). Sexual assault and physical health: Findings from a population-based study of older adults. *Psychosomatic Medicine, 62*, 838–843.

Stein, M.B., Yehuda, R., Koverola, C., and Hanna, C. (1997). Enhanced dexamethasone suppression of plasma cortisol in adult women traumatized by childhood sexual abuse. *Biological Psychiatry, 42*, 680–686.

Stone, A., Reed, B., and Neale, J. (1987). Changes in daily event frequency precede episodes of physical symptoms. *Journal of Human Stress, 13*(2), 70–74.

Talley, N.J., Fett, S.L., and Zinsmeister, A.R. (1995). Self-reported abuse and gastrointestinal disease in outpatients: Association with irritable bowel-type symptoms. *American Journal of Gastroenterology, 90*, 366–371.

Thakkar, R., and McCanne, T. (2000). The effects of daily stressors on physical health in women with and without a childhood history of sexual abuse. *Child Abuse and Neglect, 24*(2), 209–221.

Thompson, M.P., Kingree, J.B., and Desai, S. (2004). Gender differences in long-term health consequences of physical abuse of children: Data from a nationally representative survey. *American Journal of Public Health, 94*(4), 599–604.

Thompson, M.P., Arias, I., Basile, K.C., and Desai, S. (2002). The association between childhood physical and sexual victimization and health problems in adulthood in a nationally representative sample of women. *Journal of Interpersonal Violence, 17*(10), 1115–1129.

Turner, H.A., and Muller, P.A. (2004). Long-term effects of child corporal punishment on depressive symptoms in young adults: Potential moderators and mediators. *Journal of Family Issues, 25*(6), 761–782.

Waldinger, R.J., Schulz, M.S., Barsky, A.J., and Ahern, D.K. (2006). Mapping the road from childhood trauma to adult somatization: The role of attachment. *Psychosomatic Medicine, 68*(1), 129–135.

Walker, E.A., Gelfand, A., Katon, J., Koss, M., Von Korff, M., Bernstein, D., *et al.* (1999). Adult health status of women with histories of childhood abuse. *American Journal of Medicine, 107*, 332–339.

Williamson, D.F., Thompson, T.J., Anda, R.F., Dietz, W.H., and Felitti, V. (2002). Body weight and obesity in adults and self-reported abuse in childhood. *International Journal of Obesity, 26*, 1075–1082.

Wilson, A.E., Calhoun, K.S., and Bernat, J.A. (1999). Risk recognition and trauma-related symptoms among sexually revictimized women. *Journal of Consulting and Clinical Psychology, 67*(5), 705–710.

Yehuda, R., Boisoneau, D., Lowy, M.T., and Giller, E.L. (1995). Dose-response changes in plasma cortisol and lymphocyte glucocorticoid receptors following dexamethasone administration in combat veterans with and without posttraumatic stress disorder. *Archives of General Psychiatry, 52*, 583–593.

Zelman, D., Howland, E., Nichols, S., and Cleeland, C. (1991). The effects of induced mood on laboratory pain. *Pain, 46*(1), 105–111.

Zuravin, S.J., and Fontanella, C. (1999). The relationship between child sexual abuse and major depression among low-income women: A function of growing up experiences? *Child Maltreatment, 4*(1), 3–12.

The role of childhood trauma in chronic pain and fatigue

Boudewijn Van Houdenhove,
Patrick Luyten, and Ulrich Tiber Egle

CHRONIC FATIGUE SYNDROME (CFS) and the related fibromyalgia (FM) syndrome are largely overlapping disorders, mainly characterized by long-lasting, medically unexplained physical and mental fatigue, effort intolerance and widespread musculoskeletal pain. Consensus diagnostic criteria have been formulated for both syndromes (Fukuda *et al.*, 1994; Wolfe *et al.*, 1990), but the definition and delineation of the syndromes remain controversial (Nimnuan *et al.*, 2001; Reeves *et al.*, 2003; Wessely and White, 2004), and even the very existence of the syndromes has been a matter of debate (Van Houdenhove, 2003).

Despite intensive research efforts, many questions with regard to the etiological determinants and pathogenetic mechanisms of the syndromes remain unresolved. Nonetheless, evidence is growing that chronic physical and/or psychosocial stress may play a predisposing, precipitating, and perpetuating role in CFS as well as in FM (Prins *et al.*, 2006; Van Houdenhove and Egle, 2004). Evidently, stress may take different forms, such as negative life events (e.g., death of a spouse, divorce), daily hassles (e.g., persistent job problems, family conflicts), or the burden of an overactive lifestyle (e.g., due to excessive perfectionism, or self-sacrificing care-giving). But besides these common stresses in adulthood, many clinicians have been struck by the high prevalence of early life stress and particularly early traumatic or victimization experiences (i.e., maltreatment, abuse, and/or neglect) in the history of CFS and FM patients (Van Houdenhove *et al.*, 2001a). During the past decades, the prevalence and long-term consequences of early life stress have been intensively studied, and it is now believed that such experiences may play an etio-pathogenetic role in many psychiatric and physical disorders in later life (Arnow, 2004; Egle *et al.*, 2005; Kendall-Tackett, 2004; McCauley *et al.*, 1995, 1997). However, systematic investigations on the possible link between early life stress and chronic pain or fatigue have not led to unequivocal conclusions. Hence, some authors plead for more investigations in this domain (Kendall-Tackett, 2001), but others warn of multiple methodological pitfalls threatening this endeavour (Raphael *et al.*, 2004; Raphael, 2005).

In this chapter, we will examine the evidence for these connections through summaries of both controlled studies on childhood trauma in FM and CFS patients, and two of our own studies in a mixed CFS/FM sample. These results help us consider the multiple and complex pathways that may lead from victimization to chronic pain and fatigue as well as methodological problems inherent of research on this topic. These issues and their implications for practice are discussed in light of both an illustrative case report and suggested connections between research findings in clinical terms, and we propose some guidelines for health care providers.

CHILDHOOD TRAUMA IN FM

Most studies on early traumatic experiences in FM patients have been published in rheumatology journals, and focused mainly on patients with a primary FM diagnosis. As shown in Table 2.1, higher frequencies of such experiences were systematically reported by patients with FM (or mixed FM/CFS) compared to organic-medical control groups, although percentages considerably differed among patients.

TABLE 2.1 Prevalence of childhood trauma (retrospective, controlled studies) in FM patients and CFS/FM patients (statistical difference in comparison with a non-abused control group)

	% of abuse survivors in patient group	p-value
Emotional neglect/abuse		
Van Houdenhove *et al.* (2001a)	48%	p<.01
Imbierowicz and Egle (2003)	52%	p<.01
Physical maltreatment		
Boisset-Pioro *et al.* (1995)	13%	p<.01
Walker *et al.* (1997)	15%	p<.01
Alexander *et al.* (1998)	28%	p<.01
Van Houdenhove *et al.* (2001a)	23%	p<.01
Imbierowicz and Egle (2003)	31%	p<.01
Sexual abuse		
Boisset-Pioro *et al.* (1995)	37%	p<.01
Taylor *et al.* (1995)	33%	p<.01
Walker *et al.* (1997)	33%	p<.01
Alexander *et al.* (1998)	57%	p<.01
Goldberg *et al.* (1999)	65%	p<.01
Van Houdenhove *et al.* (2001a)	10%	n.s.
Imbierowicz and Egle (2003)	11%	p<.05

Davis *et al.* (2005) recently analysed controlled studies concerning a possible relationship between childhood trauma and chronic pain, including FM. The authors summarize their results as follows: (1) *individuals* reporting a history of abuse or neglect also report more pain and related symptoms compared to individuals without such a history; (2) *patients* with chronic pain report more abuse or neglect in childhood compared to healthy controls; (3) *patients* with chronic pain report more abuse or neglect than chronic pain sufferers *in the community*; and (4) people in the community suffering from chronic pain report more abuse or neglect compared to *pain-free* individuals.

Taken together, this meta-analysis clearly confirms that people who have experienced a traumatic childhood are more at risk for chronic pain in adulthood than those without such a history.

CHILDHOOD TRAUMA IN CFS

Although many clinicians have observed a high prevalence of emotional neglect or abuse, and physical or sexual trauma in CFS patients (Cuykx *et al.*, 1998; Ware and Kleinman, 1992), systematic research in this domain is still scarce. Yet, evidence for a link between childhood trauma and chronic fatigue is growing based on investigations in selected samples as well as community samples (Fisher and Chalder, 2003; Romans *et al.*, 2002).

Recently, a methodologically sophisticated population-based case-control study has been carried out on 43 individuals with CFS compared to 60 non-fatigued controls (Heim *et al.*, 2006). CFS cases reported significantly higher levels of early traumatic experiences (abuse, maltreatment, and/or neglect) and psychopathology compared to controls; exposure to childhood trauma was associated with three- to eight-fold increased risk for CFS across different trauma types; and there was a graded relationship between the degree of trauma exposure and CFS risk. Childhood trauma was also associated with greater CFS symptom severity. In addition, symptoms of depression, anxiety, and posttraumatic stress disorder were also higher for those exposed to trauma. This is significant because the risk of CFS conveyed by childhood trauma increased with the presence of concurrent psychopathology.

The authors concluded that childhood trauma is an important risk factor for CFS and that this risk was, in part, associated with altered emotional state. Although further studies are needed to replicate these findings, they add to the existing retrospective evidence that an important subset of CFS patients suffered from severe life stress during childhood.

OUR RESEARCH: CHILDHOOD TRAUMA IN CFS/FM

CONTROLLED PREVALENCE STUDY

Taking account of the large overlap between both syndromes (Aaron *et al.*, 2000), our research group carried out two studies on a mixed sample of patients with either a CFS and/or FM diagnosis. We first tried to answer the question whether childhood victimization experiences were more prevalent and more severe in these patients – seen in a tertiary university clinic setting – as compared to medical and healthy control groups (Van Houdenhove *et al.*, 2001a).

Victimization was assessed by a Dutch self-report questionnaire on burdening experiences (*Vragenlijst naar Belastende Ervaringen* (VBE); Nijenhuis *et al.*, 2002) containing 26 items focusing on *emotional neglect* (for example, as a child having to take the role of an absent or sick parent), *emotional abuse* (for example, having been bullied, mobbed or stalked), *physical maltreatment* (for example, having been frequently beaten up by a parent), and *sexual abuse* (physical contact or verbal harassment). Patients could also indicate the degree they were emotionally impacted by these experiences. We also assessed later victimization throughout adult life.

We found that out of a group of 95 CFS/FM patients (mostly females), 64 percent reported at least one type of childhood and/or adult traumatic experience, compared to 42 percent of a chronic disease control group, and 49 percent of a healthy control group. The emotional impact of the victimization was also significantly higher in the patient group than in both control groups.

An even more remarkable finding in this study was that a large subgroup of patients (39 percent) reported victimization experiences during childhood and adulthood, i.e., they actually reported *lifelong* victimization. Another interesting finding was the high prevalence of emotional neglect (49 percent), emotional abuse (38 percent), and physical abuse (23 percent) as compared to the rather low prevalence of (severe) sexual abuse (10 percent).

Taken together, our findings suggested that many CFS/FM patients remained, from their early years on, entangled in burdening, threatening, or chaotic family relationships, characterized by a lack of parental care and emotional warmth, excessive demands, and the absence of limits (Repetti *et al.*, 2002).

VICTIMIZED VS. NON-VICTIMIZED PATIENTS

In a second study, we examined a larger sample of 199 patients (158 females and 42 males) with a diagnosis of CFS and/or FM, and compared victimized and non-victimized subgroups assessed by the VBE (Nijenhuis *et al.*, 2002; Van Houdenhove *et al.*, unpublished manuscript). More particularly, we compared both subgroups with respect to psychopathology using the Dutch version of the *Symptom Checklist* (*SCL-90*; Arrindell and Ettema, 1991), and with respect to several medical parameters using clinical data as well as the *Multidimensional Fatigue Index (MFI*; Smets *et al.*, 1995) and the Dutch version of the *Arthritis Impact Measurement Scale (AIMS*; Taal *et al.*, 1989).

First, we observed that victimized CFS/FM patients (N = 119) had a higher mean number of physical symptoms than their non-victimized counterparts. This is in accordance with prior findings that in patients with "functional somatic disorders" the number of symptoms was the best predictor of those who had and had not experienced childhood abuse (Katon *et al.*, 2001).

Victimized CFS/FM patients further showed significantly higher scores on several psychopathology variables, i.e., depressive mood, inadequacy, interpersonal sensitivity and hostility, as well as on total psychoneuroticism (Table 2.2).

TABLE 2.2 Comparison between the victimized and non-victimized CFS/FM subgroups on the *SCL-90*

	Victimized	Non-victimized	p
Anxiety	23.27	20.77	n.s.
Agoraphobia	12.21	10.82	n.s.
Depression	41.94	35.24	<0.01
Somatization	35.65	33.76	n.s.
Inadequacy	25.87	23.67	<0.05
Interpersonal sensitivity	39.17	31.21	<0.01
Hostility	10.81	9.41	<0.01
Sleep difficulties	8.41	8.20	n.s.
Psychoneuroticism	215.48	187.74	<0.01

0.05 is considered significant and 0.01 is considered highly significant.

With regard to fatigue, victimized CFS/FM patients reported generally higher symptom levels and emphasized different dimensions of fatigue. In particular, impairment of mental functioning, as well as lack of activity and motivation were more prominent in this subgroup (Table 2.3). On the other hand, victimized versus non-victimized subgroups showed little difference with respect to pain measures, including the number of tender points (Table 2.3). However, patients with a history of physical abuse did report more pain (data not shown).

TABLE 2.3 Comparison of the victimized and non-victimized CFS/FM subgroups on the MFI and the AIMS

	Victimized	Non-victimized	p
MFI*			
General fatigue	18.63	17.50	<0.01
Physical fatigue	17.48	16.70	n.s.
Mental fatigue	13.78	12.41	<0.05
Reduced motivation	15.25	13.90	<0.05
Reduced activity	15.25	13.90	<0.05
Fatigue index	78.40	72.00	<0.01

Note
*higher score means more disturbance

AIMS*			
Pain	3.89	4.30	n.s.
Mobility	7.42	8.40	<0.01
Physical activity	3.56	4.03	n.s.
Social activity	4.39	4.85	n.s.
Household	8.59	8.76	n.s.
Dexterity	7.68	8.38	<0.05
ADL	9.62	9.81	n.s.
Anxiety	4.18	4.62	n.s.
Depression	4.81	5.52	<0.01
Importance of health	4.60	5.00	n.s.
Impact	2.94	3.06	n.s.

Note
*lower score means more disturbance

Overall, these results suggest that victimized CFS/FM patients suffer more psychologically and physically compared to their non-victimized counterparts. Our data with regard to pain add to inconsistent findings in prior studies, some of which showed a link between traumatic experiences, pain, and psychological distress (Alexander *et al.*, 1998; McBeth *et al.*, 1999; Walker *et al.*, 1997), while others did not (Aaron *et al.*, 1997).

CRITIQUES OF PREVIOUS APPROACHES

A MODEST RELATIONSHIP?

In an introduction to a special issue of the *Clinical Journal of Pain*, Raphael (2005) states that the relationship between childhood abuse and chronic pain, if any, should be considered "modest." To support her view, the author put forward the following arguments, on which we will critically comment:

1 The above meta-analysis (Davis *et al.*, 2005) shows rather small effect sizes in terms of Cohen's criteria (Cohen, 1988). In fact, the largest effect size found in the comparison of pain symptoms between abused and non-abused groups was only 0.33, which raises doubts about the etiological and clinical relevance of the abuse-pain relationship. [*Comment*: For disorders such as chronic pain that are based on a complex interaction of biological and psychosocial factors, effect sizes of a single risk factor are unlikely to be more substantial. Indeed, a number of recent discussions about effect size point to the complexity of determining the practical importance of effect sizes and note instances when small numeric effect sizes may have important practice and policy implications (e.g., McCartney and Rosenthal, 2000; Prentice and Miller, 1992).]

2 Nearly all childhood abuse data are based on retrospective reports implying the possibility of *recall bias*. For example, a court-documented prospective sexual/physical abuse study on FM patients did *not*

confirm retrospective data (Raphael *et al.*, 2002) and, likewise, a recent study on chronic pain patients showed discrepant findings between self-reported and *documented* sexual abuse (Brown *et al.*, 2005). On the other hand, the relationship between self-reported abuse and adult back pain was supported by two prospective cohort studies (Kopec and Sayre, 2005; Linton, 2002). [*Comment*: Authoritative reviewers emphasize that discrepancies between retrospective recall and documented abuse do not necessarily point to the unreliability of self-report. Indeed, many instances of abuse are not legally documented, and about one-third of adults with documented childhood abuse do not report about it in follow-up studies (Brewin *et al.*, 1993; Hardt and Rutter, 2004).]

3 The question may be raised to what extent abuse reports are influenced by current emotions, for example, depressive mood at the time of reporting (reporting bias). [*Comment*: It was recently shown that the abuse–pain relationship remained significant after controlling for current psychological status (Brown *et al.*, 2005). This finding is consistent with former research showing that mood in general has little influence on retrospective reports of childhood events (Brewin *et al.*, 1993).]

4 Another question is to what extent personal interpretation of a traumatic event may play a role in some types of reported abuse (*interpretation bias*). [*Comment*: This may be particularly the case in reports of emotional neglect or even physical maltreatment, but probably much less so in reports of severe or more "objective" traumatic events such as rape or the death of a close relative (Ciccone *et al.*, 2005; Hardt and Rutter, 2004).]

5 The majority of studies showing a link between childhood abuse and chronic pain have been carried out in patients who seek help, and mostly in tertiary care

settings. This may raise the possibility of *selection bias*,
meaning that a history of abuse (or associated emotional
problems such as depression or posttraumatic stress
disorder) could merely be a risk for health care seeking.
In other words, studies from selected patient groups may
give an exaggerated picture of the prevalence of a
traumatic history among chronic pain patients.
[*Comment*: The population-based CFS study by Heim
et al., 2006), discussed earlier, suggests that selection
bias may not be as important as is sometimes assumed,
but further research is needed to address this issue.]

A MORE NUANCED PICTURE
Taking the above arguments together, the skepticism of some
authors about the evidence regarding the relationship between
childhood trauma and chronic pain/fatigue seems
understandable (Morley, 2004; Raphael *et al.*, 2004; Raphael,
2005; Taylor and Jason, 2001, 2002). Nonetheless, a more
nuanced picture may emerge when interpreting the existing
research against the following background:

1 Chronic pain and fatigue patients are an etiologically
  heterogeneous group, implying that childhood trauma
  neither plays a *specific* nor a *necessary* etiological role in
  these conditions. Clearly, not all CFS/FM patients report
  such experiences, and many patients with other disorders
  report early life stress as well (Alexander *et al.*, 1998;
  Finestone *et al.*, 2000; Van Houdenhove *et al.*, 2001b).
2 The way victimization is assessed may play a crucial role in
  prevalence studies. For example, large-scale population
  studies are free from selection bias but, on the other
  hand, are usually limited to the assessment of manifest
  sexual and physical abuse (Raphael *et al.*, 2002; Taylor and
  Jason, 2001, 2002). Moreover, such studies often use brief
  telephone interviews (Ciccone *et al.*, 2005) which
  precludes the detection of more subtle forms of
  victimization, such as parental depression or drug abuse,

emotional neglect, continuous verbal humiliation, tyrannical overprotection, and so on; Kinzl *et al.*, 1995; Van Houdenhove and Egle, 2002; Wind and Silvern, 1994). A tendency to underreport childhood traumatic events is even likely to play a role in studies using extended interviews since, as noted above, many individuals seem to have forgotten these events or refuse to discuss them because of social desirability and/or shame (Brewin *et al.*, 1993; Hardt and Rutter, 2004).

3 Childhood and adult adversities may interact with other vulnerability factors (e.g., physical ailments or cognitive deficiencies) as well as protective factors (e.g., social or legal support, or intellectual or athletic capacities) which could explain why the predictive value of a traumatic history for adult chronic pain has been difficult to demonstrate prospectively (Van Houdenhove and Egle, 2002). We would add that, as our knowledge of the interplay between vulnerability and resilience increases (Charney, 2004; Southwick *et al.*, 2005), the effect of childhood victimization on later development should not be understood in terms of a direct, linear, and all-or-none fashion, but in the context of complex, reciprocal, and probabilistic interactions between various biological and psychosocial factors (Luyten *et al.*, 2006).

4 The fact that modern neurobiological research has provided "hard" evidence for the etiological role of early adverse experiences in various mental and physical disorders during later life makes the contribution of such experiences in chronic pain and fatigue increasingly plausible (see also point 5).

5 Finally, whereas more prospective, community-based research in this domain is undoubtedly needed, methodologically sophisticated retrospective studies in well-defined patient groups may still provide useful information (Hardt and Rutter, 2004; Heim *et al.*, 2006; Kendall-Tackett and Becker-Blease, 2004). In particular,

retrospective studies may be better able to capture the chronic, multiple, and often subtle traumatic situations that characterize the history of an important subset of CFS/FM patients (Van Houdenhove *et al.*, 2001a; Van Houdenhove and Egle, 2002).

FROM VICTIMIZATION TO CHRONIC PAIN/FATIGUE
What do we know about the *mechanisms* linking childhood trauma with CFS/FM? A complex interaction of psychological factors and physiological mechanisms seems to play a role, the relative importance of which may be different in each patient (Kendall-Tackett, 2002). Early traumatic experiences may influence personality traits such as neuroticism or negative affectivity, which are known to increase somatization tendencies (Talley *et al.*, 1998). Within attachment theory, these traits may be considered to be the result of insecure or disorganized attachment (Chiechanowski *et al.*, 2002, 2003; Mikail *et al.*, 1994).

A number of psychophysiological mechanisms could explain *how* such personality factors may facilitate chronic fatigue and pain, for example, by causing high sympathetic arousal (which may be exhausting in the long term), long-lasting sleep problems (which may impair recovery), muscle hypertension and chronic hyperventilation (which may increase muscle pain), hypervigilance for physical stimuli (which may augment symptom perception), and possibly also altered pain processing (Fillingham and Edwards, 2005; Scarinci *et al.*, 1994).

Victimized individuals are as a rule characterized by less effective psychological defense and coping styles, which may lead to increased sensitivity for future stressors and also imply unhealthy behaviors and lifestyle (such as excessive drinking, eating, or smoking), exaggerated health care seeking (carrying the risk of medical overconsumption, iatrogenic complications, and increased disability), as well as psychiatric problems such as anxiety, depression, and sleep disorders. All these factors may directly or indirectly contribute to the patient's pain, fatigue, and other symptoms, and worsen functional limitations (Lampe *et al.*, 2003; Nickel and Egle, 2006).

The relationship between childhood trauma and chronic pain and fatigue could also be mediated by neuroendocrine mechanisms. In this respect, pioneering animal research has suggested that early adverse experiences may dramatically impact the development of the stress system, causing impaired stress tolerance in later life (Insel and Young, 2001). More concretely, it has been demonstrated that the quality of maternal care may influence gene expression of vital components of the stress system, such as the hippocampal glucocorticoid receptor that plays a crucial role in "containing" and adequately finishing the stress response (McEwen, 2003; McEwen and Lasley, 2002; Meaney, 2001). In addition, human studies have shown that the quality of mother-child attachment may largely determine the way the person will create his or her own environment and perceive life stresses and adversities, which may in turn have profound neurobiological effects (Gunnar, 2003).

Thus, one could assume that childhood trauma, in interaction with genetic factors (for example, 5-HT transporter gene polymorphism; see Offenbaecher *et al.*, 1999), may make the developing child's stress-response system more vulnerable for the dysregulating effects of subsequent acute or chronic stressors, such as later maltreatment by an abusive partner or the chronic burden of an overactive lifestyle, which in victimized individuals often serve the purpose of regulating inner tension and restlessness, compensating for low self-esteem (Van Houdenhove, 2002).

Retrospective as well as prospective human studies are now beginning to explore the complex pathways along which consequences of adverse childhood experiences may co-determine various aspects of psychological as well as physical adult health (Anda *et al.*, 2006; Batten *et al.*, 2004; Felitti *et al.*, 1998; Goodwin and Stein, 2004; Russek and Schwartz, 1997). In particular, HPA-axis dysregulation – hyper(re)activity as well as hypo(re)activity – has been found to be associated with childhood trauma and may be considered an important vulnerability factor for stress-related psychiatric and physical disorders (Gunnar and Vazquez, 2001; Heim *et al.*, 2000, 2002; Heim and Nemeroff, 2001; Van Voorhees and Scarpa, 2004).

In this context, more studies should be undertaken that shed light on the specific neurobiological mechanisms by which victimized individuals might be more prone to chronic pain and fatigue. As an example of such studies, it was recently found that FM patients with a history of childhood abuse had disturbed morning cortisol levels and flattened diurnal salivary cortisol rhythms (McLean *et al.*, 2005; Weisbecker *et al.*, 2006; see also Luyten and Van Houdenhove, 2006). In another study on HPA-axis functioning it was demonstrated that CFS patients reporting a traumatic history differed significantly from their non-abused counterparts with regard to basal cortisol levels as well as cortisol suppression using the dexamethason/CRH test (Van Den Eede *et al.*, 2008).

CASE REPORT

Examination of individual cases in which these variables co-occur can be instructive in suggesting next steps for research and practice. In this section we present the case of one individual who illustrates the links between fibromyalgia and a history of traumatic experiences with special attention to points of intervention.

A 44-year-old woman, employed as a commercial assistant, developed pain in the low back and temporo-mandibular region during the period of her divorce. She had been married to a man who was pathologically jealous, had a serious alcohol problem, and regularly maltreated her. Orthopaedic and dental treatments (including the extraction of two healthy teeth) did not bring any amelioration. A proposal for lumbar surgery was refused by the patient. During the following two years, her pain became more and more generalized. One year after the divorce, the patient's only daughter, with whom she had a very close relationship, left home for college.

After consulting a rheumatologist, she was diagnosed with fibromyalgia (FM). Two hospitalizations on a rheumatological ward resulted in some temporary pain decrease. Meanwhile, the patient had lost her job owing to regular sickness absences. The only positive thing in her life was that she had met a new partner whom she remarried shortly thereafter. This man showed much understanding and emotional warmth toward her, but she lived in constant fear that he would leave her.

Eight years after the onset of her pain – during which she consulted 14 different physicians – she eventually attended a university psychosomatic clinic. Here it was concluded that she suffered from chronic widespread pain in the context of dysthymia and a personality disorder.

The patient's biography revealed long-standing sexual abuse by her alcohol-dependent stepfather from the age of 7 to 10. Her mother apparently knew about the abusive contacts, but didn't do anything about it. Moreover, the patient was regularly physically maltreated by her older brother, and witnessed the frequent violent fights between her parents. Her younger sister was also abused by her stepfather, and when this girl attempted to warn her mother about what was happening, she encountered disbelief and was called a liar. Promptly thereafter, she began bed-wetting again, and was declared "retarded" and "mad" by the parents. The patient herself firmly resolved to keep the abuse secret and "grin and bear it."

Already as a child she was very inhibited and fearful, and completely lacked self-confidence. She often had headaches, diarrhea, and stomach pains, was suspected of appendicitis and, at age 14, eventually underwent an appendectomy.

When at age 17 she met her first husband, she was impressed by his self-reliant attitude, and she married him one year later. Soon, however, she discovered that he was a severe alcoholic with an impulsive and aggressive character.

In the psychosomatic clinic, she had the opportunity to attend a psychodynamic-interactional, manualized group therapy on an ambulatory basis for six months. An antidepressant (sertraline

50 mg), and low-level fitness training were also added to her therapeutic program. Meanwhile, she had found a new (part-time) job, which was sufficiently adapted to her functional limitations.

A central theme in the group therapy was her low self-esteem that negatively interfered with her marital relationship and social interactions. From this perspective, initial therapeutic interventions often focused on her wish to be "a perfect patient." She became more aware of her fears of abandonment and rejection, and succeeded in working through these fears in the group-dynamic process and subsequently in her family and job environment. These success experiences encouraged her to progressively take her own needs and interests more into account, particularly in her new job. Positive reactions from her husband and colleagues fostered her trust in other people, and stimulated her to pursue a more satisfying way of interacting with others and enjoying life.

At the end of the therapy, the patient was nearly pain-free without any medication. Only occasional "memories about the past" could again trigger a short pain increase but without provoking "catastrophizing" thoughts. At the one-year follow-up, it appeared that she still suffered from time to time from pain in the left hip, but this localized pain didn't bother her too much in her daily activities. The relationship with her husband became more emotionally intense. Her fears of loss disappeared, and she felt appreciated and recognized in her job, and her nightly bruxism became more rare. "In fact, I feel happy for the first time in my life," she confided to her therapist during the final follow-up consultation.

CLINICAL IMPLICATIONS

No doubt, CFS/FM patients with a history of abuse or neglect are a great challenge for their doctors or other health care providers. Some of these patients suffer from full-blown posttraumatic stress disorder, or – more commonly – show sub-threshold posttraumatic stress symptoms, which require a specific therapeutic approach (Ciccone *et al.*, 2005; Raphael, 2005; Van Houdenhove, 2006a).

Moreover, as mentioned before, these patients may bear the negative consequences of insecure or disorganized attachment, leading to personality disturbances such as borderline personality disorder (Battle *et al.*, 2004; Chiechanowski *et al.*, 2002; Goodman *et al.*, 2004; Mikail *et al.*, 1994), which may make relationships with caregivers ambiguous or even overtly conflictual (Stuart and Noyes, 1999).

Consequently, health care professionals should take these potential difficulties into account and, therefore, tactfully question CFS/FM patients about childhood adversities (Van Houdenhove, 2006b). For example, one could say: "I would like to know somewhat more about you as a child. How was the family atmosphere at home? How was the mutual understanding between your parents, and between you and your brothers and sisters? Was there someone who used to drink too much alcohol, used drugs, or was physically violent? Did someone in your family have long-standing mental problems? Did your parents show understanding and support you when you were worrying about something or had emotional difficulties? Was your privacy respected at home? Have you been bullied at school? Have you ever been a victim of physical assault, or been forced to do sexual things?"

Primary care physicians, in particular, are in a good position to assess victimization experiences in the context of a biopsychosocial diagnostic evaluation. Since they usually have a close and trusting relationship with the patient, questions about life history and family context are mostly well accepted. Health care professionals should overcome fears of offending patients by asking such questions, since most patients feel comfortable discussing their life history and consider it relevant to their medical care (Meagher, 2004).

Although cognitive behaviour therapy (CBT) and progressive, low-level exercise training have proven to be useful for many CFS/FM patients (Goldenberg *et al.*, 2004; Prins *et al.*, 2006), a substantial subgroup does not respond very well to these, or drops out prematurely from these therapies. Non-responders or drop-outs typically show a low baseline physical activity level, a passive coping style, and a lack of self-efficacy (Prins *et al.*, 2005; Van der Werf *et al.*, 2000). We believe that such characteristics may, in many cases, be linked to early traumatic experiences. These experiences may in turn lead to more physical and psychological suffering, including affective comorbidity, but may also increase the risk of inadequate illness behavior based on immature psychological defense styles (Nickel and Egle, 2006).

Consequently, we suggest that this subgroup of CFS/FM patients would need a modified, more comprehensive therapeutic approach – comparable to what has been proposed for other victimized patients (see, e.g., Craighead and Nemeroff, 2005). To that aim, principles and strategies of "dialectic behaviour therapy" (Linehan, 1993), "emotion focused therapy" (Greenberg and Paivio, 1997), or "schema focused therapy" (Young *et al.*, 2003) could be built into the CBT-treatment protocol. Generally, patients who suffer severe sequelae from early life trauma also need longer term therapy – as the above case report illustrates. But, unfortunately, studies testing such extended treatment approaches are currently lacking. In addition, future research should investigate the relative efficacy and effectiveness of different treatment regimens for different subsets of patients, especially CFS/FM patients with a traumatic history (Luyten and Van Houdenhove, in press).

For those CFS/FM patients who are severely incapacitated mentally and/or physically, a day clinic or residential (group) setting would be indicated. Such a treatment setting may represent a "holding environment" in which a trustful therapeutic alliance can develop, resistances and transference reactions are sensitively handled, and the patients' motivation for active coping progressively fostered. Such a setting may also allow to integrate CBT and graded exercise training with experiential, psychodynamic or interpersonal strategies, and combine them with mind–body-oriented psychomotor and creative therapeutic techniques, as well as rational psychopharmacotherapy to correct affective comorbidity (Cuykx *et al.*, 1998; Essame *et al.*, 1998; Van Houdenhove, 2002).

In this way, victimized CFS/FM patients could gradually ameliorate their problem-solving capacities using more mature defense styles, resolve energy-consuming intra- and interpersonal conflicts, more adequately regulate positive and negative emotions, engage in a more balanced lifestyle, realistically adjust life goals, and succeed in optimal and long-term self-care.

CONCLUSIONS

Evidence is growing that childhood trauma may be an important vulnerability factor for "unexplained" chronic pain and fatigue. Not only have studies demonstrated that chronic pain patients and, more particularly, CFS/FM patients frequently report early traumatic experiences. Neurobiological investigations have also made increasingly plausible that such experiences may have a dramatic impact on the development of the stress system – and consequently on the proneness to various stress- and lifestyle-related disorders, including CFS/FM. Yet, researchers in this field should be aware of many methodological pitfalls that may bias childhood trauma studies and, thus, should refrain from premature conclusions.

Nonetheless, clinical wisdom and existing research data suggest that victimized CFS/FM patients may be best considered a distinct subgroup, with different symptomatic and functional characteristics, and different therapeutic needs. Further controlled investigations should find out whether a more specific and comprehensive therapeutic approach – as proposed in this chapter – could lead to a better outcome for these patients.

REFERENCES

Aaron, L.A., Burke, M.M., and Buchwald, D. (2000). Overlapping conditions among patients with chronic fatigue syndrome, fibromyalgia, and temporomandibular disorder. *Archives of Internal Medicine, 24,* 221–227.

Aaron, L.A., Bradley, L.A., Alarcon, G.S., Triana-Alexander, M., Alexander, R.W., Martin, M.Y., *et al.* (1997). Perceived physical and emotional trauma as precipitating events in fibromyalgia. Associations with health care seeking and disability status but not pain severity. *Arthritis and Rheumatism, 40,* 453–460.

Alexander, R.W., Bradley, L.A., Alarcon, G.S., Triana-Alexander, M., Aaron, L.A., Alberts, K.R., *et al.* (1998). Sexual and physical abuse in women with fibromyalgia: Associations with outpatient healthcare utilisation and main medication usage. *Arthritis Care* and *Research, 11,* 102–115.

Anda, R.F., Felitti, V.J., Bremner, J.D., Walker, J.D., Whitfield, C., Perry, B.D., *et al.* (2006). The enduring effects of abuse and related adverse experiences in childhood. A convergence of evidence from neurobiology and epidemiology. *European Archives of Psychiatry and Clinical Neuroscience, 256,* 174–186.

Arnow, B.A. (2004). Relationships between childhood maltreatment, adult health and psychiatric outcomes, and medical utilization. *Journal of Clinical Psychiatry, 65* (Suppl 12), 10–15.

Arrindell, W.A., and Ettema, J.M.H. (1991). *Handleiding bij een multidimensionele psychopathologie-indicator.* Lisse: Swets & Zeitlinger.

Batten, S.V., Aslan, M., Maciejewski, P.K., and Mazure, C.M. (2004). Childhood maltreatment as a risk factor for adult cardiovascular disease and depression. *Journal of Clinical Psychiatry, 65,* 249–254.

Battle, C.L., Shea, M.T., Johnson, D.M., Yen, S., Zlotnick, C., Zanarini, M.C., *et al.* (2004). Childhood maltreatment associated with adult personality disorder: Findings from the Collaborative Longitudinal Personality Disorders Study. *Journal of Personality Disorders, 18,* 193–211.

Boisset-Pioro, M.H., Esdaile, J.M., and Fitzcharles, M.A. (1995). Sexual and physical abuse in women with fibromyalgia syndrome. *Arthritis and Rheumatism, 38,* 235–241.

Brewin, C.R., Andrews, B., and Gotlib, I.H. (1993). Psychopathology and early experience: A reappraisal of retrospective reports. *Psychological Bulletin, 113,* 82–98.

Brown, J., Berenson, K., and Cohen, P. (2005). Documented and self-reported child abuse and adult pain in a community sample. *Clinical Journal of Pain, 21,* 374–377.

Charney, D.S. (2004). Psychobiological mechanisms of resilience and vulnerability: Implications for successful adaptation to extreme stress. *American Journal of Psychiatry, 161,* 195–216.

Chiechanowski, P., Katon, W.J., Russo, J.E., and Dwight-Johnson, M.M. (2002). Association of attachment style to lifetime medically unexplained symptoms in patients with hepatitis C. *Psychosomatics, 43*, 206–312.

Chiechanowski, P., Sullivan, M., Jensen, M., Romano, J., and Summers, H. (2003). The relationship of attachment style to depression, catastrophizing and health care utilization in patients with chronic pain. *Pain, 104*, 627–637.

Ciccone, D.S., Elliott, D.K., Chandler, H.K., Nayak, S., and Raphael, K.G. (2005). Sexual and physical abuse in women with fibromyalgia syndrome. A test of the trauma hypothesis. *Clinical Journal of Pain, 21*, 378–386.

Cohen, J. (1988). *Statistical power analysis for the behavioural sciences* (2nd edn). New York: Academic Press.

Craighead, W.E., and Nemeroff, C.B. (2005). The impact of early trauma on response to psychotherapy. *Clinical Neuroscience Research, 4*, 405–411.

Cuykx, V., Van Houdenhove, B., and Neerinckx, E. (1998). Childhood abuse, personality disorder, and chronic fatigue syndrome. *General Hospital Psychiatry, 20*, 382–384.

Davis, D.A., Luecken, L.J., and Zautra, A.J. (2005). Are reports of childhood abuse related to the experience of chronic pain in adulthood? A meta-analytic review of the literature. *Clinical Journal of Pain, 21*, 398–405.

Egle, U.T., Hoffmann, S.O., and Joraschky, P. (eds) (2005). *Sexueller missbrauch, misshandlung, vernachlässigung*. Stuttgart/New York: Schattauer.

Essame, C.S., Ohelan, S., Aggett, P., and White, P.D. (1998). Pilot study of a multidisciplinary inpatient rehabilitation of severe incapacitated patients with the chronic fatigue syndrome. *Journal of Chronic Fatigue Syndrome, 4*, 51–58.

Felitti, V.J., Anda, R.F., Nordenberg, D., Williamson, D.F., Spitz, A.M., Edwards, V., *et al.* (1998). Relationship of childhood abuse and household dysfunction to many of the leading causes of death in adults. The Adverse Childhood Experiences (ACE) Study. *American Journal of Preventive Medicine, 14*, 245–258.

Fillingim, R.B., and Edwards, R.R. (2005). Is self-reported childhood abuse history associated with pain perception among healthy young women and men? *Clinical Journal of Pain, 21*, 367–397.

Finestone, H.M., Stenn, P., Davies, F., Stalker, C., Fry, R., and Koumaris, J. (2000). Chronic pain and health care utilisation in women with a history of childhood sexual abuse. *Child Abuse and Neglect, 24*, 547–556.

Fisher, L., and Chalder, T. (2003). Childhood experiences of illness and parenting in adults with chronic fatigue syndrome. *Journal of Psychosomatic Research, 54*, 439–443.

Fukuda, K., Straus, S., Hickie, I., Sharpe, M., Dobbins, J., and Komaroff, A. (1994). The chronic fatigue syndrome: A comprehensive approach to its definition and study. *Annals of Internal Medicine, 121*, 953–959.

Goldberg, R.T., Pachas, W.N., and Keith, D. (1999). Relationship between traumatic events in childhood and chronic pain. *Disability and Rehabilitation, 21*, 23–30.

Goldenberg, D.L., Burckhardt, C.S., and Crofford, L. (2004). Management of fibromyalgia syndrome. *Journal of the American Medical Association, 292*, 2388–2395.

Goodman, M., New, A., and Siever, L. (2004). Trauma, genes, and the neurobiology of personality disorders. *Annals of the New York Academy of Science, 1032*, 104–116.

Goodwin, R.D., and Stein, M.B. (2004). Association between childhood trauma and physical disorder among adults in the United States. *Psychological Medicine, 34*, 509–520.

Greenberg, L.S., and Paivio, S.C. (1997). *Working with the emotions in psychotherapy*. New York: Guilford Press.

Gunnar, M.R. (2003). Integrating neuroscience and psychological approaches in the study of early experiences. *Annals of the New York Academy of Sciences, 1008*, 238–247.

Gunnar, M.R., and Vazquez, D.M. (2001). Low cortisol and flattening of expected daytime rhythm: Potential indices of risk in human development. *Developmental Psychobiology, 13*, 515–538.

Hardt, J., and Rutter, M. (2004). Validity of adult retrospective reports of adverse childhood experiences: Review of the evidence. *Journal of Child Psychology and Psychiatry, 45*, 260–273.

Heim, C., and Nemeroff, C.B. (2001). The role of childhood trauma in the neurobiology of mood and anxiety disorders: Preclinical and clinical studies. *Biological Psychiatry, 49*, 1023–1039.

Heim, C., Ehlert, U., and Hellhammer, D.H. (2000). The potential role of hypocortisolism in the pathophysiology of stress-related bodily disorders. *Psychoneuroendocrinology, 25*, 1–35.

Heim, C., Newport, D.J., Wagner, D., Wilcox, M.M, and Nemeroff, C.B. (2002). The role of early adverse experience and adult stress in the prediction of neuroendocrine stress reactivity in women: A multiple regression analysis. *Depression and Anxiety, 15*, 117–125.

Heim, C., Wagner, D., Maloney, E., Papanicolaou, D.A, Solomon, L., Jones, J.F., *et al.* (2006). Early adverse experience and risk for chronic fatigue syndrome: Results from a population-based study. *Archives of General Psychiatry, 63*, 1258–1266.

Imbierowics, K., and Egle, U.T. (2003). Childhood adversities in patients with fibromyalgia and somatoform pain disorder. *European Journal of Pain, 7*, 113–119.

Insel, T.R., and Young, L.J. (2001). The neurobiology of attachment. *Nature Reviews Neuroscience, 2*, 129–136.

Katon, W., Sullivan, M., and Walker, E. (2001). Medical symptoms without identified pathology: Relationship to psychiatric disorders, childhood and adult trauma, and personality traits. *Annals of Internal Medicine, 134*, 917–925.

Kendall-Tackett, K.A. (2001). Chronic pain: The next frontier in child maltreatment research. *Child Abuse and Neglect, 25*, 997–1000.

Kendall-Tackett, K.A. (2002). The health effects of childhood abuse: Four pathways by which abuse can influence health. *Child Abuse and Neglect, 26*, 715–729.

Kendall-Tackett, K.A. (ed.) (2004). *Health consequences of abuse in the family. A clinical guide for evidence-based practice*. Washington, DC: American Psychological Association.

Kendall-Tackett, K., and Becker-Blease, K. (2004). The importance of retrospective findings in child maltreatment research. *Child Abuse and Neglect, 28*, 723–727.

Kinzl, J.F., Traweger, C., and Biebl, W. (1995). Family background and sexual abuse associated with somatization. *Psychotherapy and Psychosomatics, 64*, 82–87.

Kopec, J.A., and Sayre, E.C. (2005). Stressful experiences in childhood and chronic back pain in the general population. *Clinical Journal of Pain, 21*, 478–483.

Lampe, A., Doering, S., Rumpold, G., Solder, E., Krismer, M., Kantner-Rumplmair, W., *et al.* (2003). Chronic pain syndromes and their relation to childhood abuse and stressful life events. *Journal of Psychosomatic Research, 54*, 361–367.

Linehan, M.M. (1993). *Cognitive-behavioral treatment of borderline personality disorder*. New York: Guilford Press.

Linton, S.J. (2002). A prospective study of the effects of sexual or physical abuse on back pain. *Pain, 96*, 347–351.

Luyten, P., and Van Houdenhove, B. (2006). Cortisol secretion and symptoms in patients with fibromyalgia: Comment on the article by McLean *et al. Arthritis and Rheumatism, 54*, 2345–2346.

Luyten, P., Blatt, S.J., Van Houdenhove, B., and Corveleyn, J. (2006). Depression research and treatment: Are we skating to where the puck is going to be? *Clinical Psychology Review, 26*, 985–999.

McBeth, J. McFarlane, G.J., Benjamin, S., Morris, S., and Silman, A.J. (1999). The association between tender points, psychological distress and adverse childhood experiences. *Arthritis and Rheumatism, 42*, 1397–1404.

McCartney, K., and Rosenthal, R. (2000). Effect size, practical importance, and social policy for children. *Child Development, 71*, 173–180.

McCauley, J., Kern, D.E., Kolodner, K., Dill, L., Schroeder, A.F., DeChant, H.K., *et al.* (1995). The battering syndrome: Prevalence and clinical characteristics of domestic violence in primary care internal medicine practices. *Annals of Internal Medicine, 123*, 737–746.

McCauley, J., Kern, D.E., Kolodner, K., Dill, L., Schroeder, A.F., DeChant, H.K., *et al.* (1997). Clinical characteristics of women with a history of childhood abuse: Unhealed wounds. *Journal of the American Medical Association, 227*, 1362–1368.

McEwen, B.S. (2003). Early life influences on life-long patterns of behavior and health. *Mental Retardation and Developmental Disabilities Research Reviews, 9*, 149–154.

McEwen, B.S., and Lasley, E. (2002). *The end of stress as we know it*. Washington, DC: Joseph Henri Press.

McLean, S.A., Williams, D.A., Harris, R.E., Kop, W.J., Groner, K.H., Ambrose, K., *et al.* (2005). Momentary relationship between cortisol secretion and symptoms in patients with fibromyalgia. *Arthritis and Rheumatism, 52*, 3660–3669.

Meagher, M.W. (2004). Links between traumatic family violence and chronic pain: Biopsychosocial pathways and treatment implications. In K.A. Kendall-Tackett (ed.), *Health consequences of abuse in the family. A clinical guide for evidence-based practice* (pp. 155–177). Washington, DC: American Psychological Association.

Meaney, M.J. (2001). Maternal care, gene expression, and the transmission of individual differences in stress reactivity across generations. *Annual Review of Neuroscience, 24,* 1161–1192.

Mikail, S.F., Henderson, P.R., and Tasca, G.A. (1994). An interpersonal based model of chronic pain: An application of attachment theory. *Clinical Psychology Review, 14,* 1–16.

Morley, S. (2004). What impact does childhood experience have on the development of chronic pain? In R.H. Dworkin and W.S. Breitbart (eds), *Psychosocial aspects of pain: A handbook for health care providers* (pp. 571–588). Seattle: IASP Press.

Nickel, R., and Egle, U.T. (2006). Psychological defense styles, childhood adversities and psychopathology in adulthood. *Child Abuse and Neglect, 30,* 157–170.

Nickel, R., Egle, U.T., and Hardt, J. (2002). Are childhood adversities relevant in patients with chronic low-back pain? *European Journal of Pain, 6,* 221–228.

Nijenhuis, E.R.S., Hart, O. van der, and Kruger, K. (2002). The psychometric characteristics of the Traumatic Experiences Checklist (TEC): First findings among psychiatric outpatients. *Clinical Psychology and Psychotherapy, 9,* 200–210.

Nimnuan, C., Rabe-Hesketh, S., Wessely, S., and Hotopf, M. (2001). How many functional somatic syndromes? *Journal of Psychosomatic Research, 51,* 549–557.

Offenbaecher, M., Bondy, B., de Jonge, S., Glatzeder, K., Kruger, M., Scheps, P., *et al.* (1999). Possible association of fibromyalgia with a polymorphism in the serotonin transporter gene regulatory region. *Arthritis and Rheumatism, 42,* 2482–2488.

Prentice, D.A. and Miller, D.T. (1992). When small effects are impressive. *Psychological Bulletin, 112,* 160–164.

Prins, J., Bleijenberg, G., Rouweler, E.K., and Van der Meer, J. (2005). Effect of psychiatric disorders on outcome of cognitive-behavioural therapy for chronic fatigue syndrome. *British Journal of Psychiatry, 187,* 184–185.

Prins, J., Van der Meer, J.W., and Bleijenberg, G. (2006). Chronic fatigue syndrome. *Lancet, 367,* 346–355.

Raphael, K.G. (2005). Childhood abuse and pain in adulthood: More than a modest relationship? *Clinical Journal of Pain, 21*, 371–373.

Raphael, K.G., Chandler, H.K., and Ciccone, D.S. (2004). Is childhood abuse a risk factor for chronic pain in adulthood? *Current Pain and Headache Reports, 8*, 99–110.

Raphael, K.G., Widom, C.S., and Lange, G. (2002). Childhood victimization and pain in adulthood: A prospective investigation. *Pain, 92*, 283–293.

Reeves, W.C., Lloyd, A., Vernon, S.D., Klimas, N., Jason, L.A., Bleijenberg, G., *et al.* (2003). International Chronic Fatigue Syndrome Study Group. Identification of ambiguities in the 1994 chronic fatigue syndrome research case definition and recommendations for resolution. *BMC Health Services Research, 3*, 25.

Repetti, L.R., Taylor, S.E., and Seeman, T.E. (2002). Risky families: Family social environments and the mental and physical health of offspring. *Psychological Bulletin, 128*, 330–366.

Romans, S., Belaise, C., Martin, J., Morris, E., and Raffi, A. (2002). Childhood abuse and later medical disorders in women. *Psychotherapy and Psychosomatics, 71*, 141–150.

Russek, L.G., and Schwartz, G.E. (1997). Perceptions of parental caring predict health status in midlife: A 35-year follow-up of the Harvard Mastery of Stress Study. *Psychosomatic Medicine, 59*, 144–149.

Scarinci, I.C., McDonald-Haile, J., Bradley, L.A., and Richter, J.E. (1994). Altered pain perception and psychosocial features among women with gastrointestinal disorders and history of abuse: a preliminary model. *American Journal of Medicine, 97*, 108–118.

Smets, E.M.A., Garsson, B., and Bonke, B. (1995). *Het meten van vermoeidheid met de multidimensionele Vermoeidheidsindex (MVI-20). Een handleiding.* Amsterdam: Medische Psychologie Academisch Centrum, Universiteit Amsterdam.

Southwick, S.M., Vythilingam, M., and Charney, D.S. (2005). The psychobiology of depression and resilience to stress: Implications for prevention and treatment. *Annual Review of Clinical Psychology, 1*, 255–291.

Stuart, S., and Noyes, R. (1999). Attachment and interpersonal communication in somatization. *Psychosomatics, 40*, 34–43.

Taal, E., Jacobs, J.W., and Seydel, E.R. (1989). Evaluation of the Dutch Arthritis Measurement Scales (Dutch-AIMS) in patients with rheumatoid arthritis. *British Journal of Rheumatology, 28*, 487–491.

Talley, N.J., Boyce, P.M., and Jones, M. (1998). Is the association between irritable bowel syndrome and abuse explained by neuroticism? A population-based study. *Gut, 42*, 47–53.

Taylor, R.R., and Jason, L.A. (2001). Sexual abuse, physical abuse, chronic fatigue, and chronic fatigue syndrome: A community-based study. *Journal of Nervous and Mental Disease, 189*, 709–715.

Taylor, R.R., and Jason, L.A. (2002). Chronic fatigue, abuse-related traumatization, and psychiatric disorders in a community-based sample. *Social Science and Medicine, 55*, 247–256.

Taylor, M.L., Trotter, D.R., and Csuka, M.E. (1995). The prevalence of sexual abuse in women with fibromyalgia. *Arthritis and Rheumatism, 38*, 229–234.

Van Den Eede F., Moorkens, G., Hulstijn, W., Van Houdenhove, B., Cosyns, P., and Sabbe, B. (2008). Combined dexamethasone/corticotropin – releasing factor test in chronic fatigue syndrome. *Psychological Medicine, 38*, 963–973.

Van der Werf, S.P., Prins, J.B., Vercoulen, J.H., Van der Meer, J.W., and Bleijenberg, G. (2000). Identifying physical activity patterns in chronic fatigue syndrome using actigraphic assessment. *Journal of Psychosomatic Research, 49*, 373–379.

Van Houdenhove, B. (2002). Listening to CFS. Why we should pay more attention to the story of the patient. *Journal of Psychosomatic Research, 52*, 495–499.

Van Houdenhove, B. (2003). Fibromyalgia: A challenge for modern medicine. *Clinical Rheumatology, 22*, 1–5.

Van Houdenhove, B. (2006a). Psychiatric comorbidity and chronic fatigue syndrome. *British Journal of Psychiatry, 188*, 395.

Van Houdenhove, B. (2006b). Assessing adverse childhood experiences in chronic pain: It does matter. *Clinical Journal of Pain, 22*, 584.

Van Houdenhove, B., and Egle, U.T. (2002). Letter to the editor. *Pain, 96*, 215–220.

Van Houdenhove, B., and Egle, U.T. (2004). Fibromyalgia: A stress disorder. Piecing the biopsychosocial puzzle together. *Psychotherapy and Psychosomatics, 73*, 267–275.

Van Houdenhove, B., and Luyten, P. (in press). Customizing treatment of chronic fatigue syndrome/fibromyalgia: The role of perpetuating factors. *Psychosomatics*.

Van Houdenhove, B., Neerinckx, E., Lysens, R., Vertommen, H., and Onghena, P. (2001b). Premorbid overactive lifestyle in chronic fatigue syndrome and fibromyalgia: An etiological factor or proof of good citizenship? *Journal of Psychosomatic Research, 51*, 571–576.

Van Houdenhove, B., Neerinckx, E., Lysens, R., Vertommen, H., Van Houdenhove, L., Onghena, P., *et al.* (2001a). Victimization in chronic fatigue syndrome and fibromyalgia in tertiary care. A controlled study on prevalence and characteristics. *Psychosomatics, 42*, 21–28.

Van Voorhees, E., and Scarpa, A. (2004). The effects of child maltreatment on the hypothalamic-pituitary-adrenal axis. *Trauma, Violence and Abuse, 5*, 333–352.

Walker, E.A., Keegan, D., Gardner, G., Sullivan, M., Bernstein, D., and Katon, W.J. (1997). Psychosocial factors in fibromyalgia compared with rheumatoid arthritis: II Sexual, physical, and emotional abuse and neglect. *Psychosomatic Medicine, 59*, 572–577.

Ware, N.C., and Kleinman, A. (1992). Culture and somatic experience: The social course of illness in neurasthenia and chronic fatigue syndrome. *Psychosomatic Medicine, 54*, 546–560.

Weisbecker, I., Floyd, A., Dedert, E., Salmon, P., and Sephton, S. (2006). Childhood trauma and diurnal disruption in fibromyalgia syndrome. *Psychoneuroendocrinology, 31*, 312–324.

Wessely, S., and White, P.D. (2004). There is only one functional somatic syndrome. *British Journal of Psychiatry, 185*, 95–96.

Wind, T.W., and Silvern, L. (1994). Parenting and family stress as mediators of the long-term effects of child abuse. *Child Abuse and Neglect, 18*, 439–453.

Wolfe, F., Smythe, H.A., Yunus, M.B., Bennett, R.M., Bombardier, C., Goldenberg, D.L., *et al.* (1990). The American College of Rheumatology 1990 criteria for the classification of fibromyalgia: Report of the multicenter criteria committee. *Arthritis and Rheumatism, 33*, 160–172.

Young, J.E., Klosko, J.S., and Weishaar, M. (2003). *Schema therapy: A practitioner's guide*. New York: Guilford Press.

The impact of traumatic childbirth on health through the undermining of breastfeeding

Cynthia Good Mojab

WOMEN'S EXPERIENCES during childbirth may range through a spectrum from challenging yet empowering to overwhelming and traumatic. Childbirth trauma is largely still an invisible issue. However, a growing literature base now documents women's possible psychological traumatization during birth (Bailham and Joseph, 2003; Declerq *et al.*, 2008; Olde *et al.*, 2006). As we understand more about the connection between birth and psychological trauma, we have also begun to recognize that these traumatic experiences can influence the initiation and continuation of breastfeeding (Kroeger and Smith, 2004; Righard and Alade, 1990; Shealy *et al.*, 2005). This link is important because there are numerous maternal and infant health risks associated with the use of artificial substitutes for human milk in the first six months of life.

Birth practices, such as the use of labor pain medications, maternal–infant separation after birth, and instrumental or operative birth, can interfere with the initiation of breastfeeding, with exclusive breastfeeding, and with the continuation of breastfeeding. Separating the impact on breastfeeding of physical trauma from that of psychological trauma is difficult.

However, to clinicians working with women who have experienced births with many technological interventions, the role of psychological trauma is clear. I am privileged to have had many women share their birth experiences with me in my counseling practice and my research. I hope that the inclusion in this chapter of some of their voices will help increase awareness of childbirth trauma and its potential to profoundly negatively impact the mother–infant dyad.

RISK FACTORS FOR TRAUMATIC BIRTH

"I emotionally separated myself from my body during the surgery. I was not there. It was like everything was happening in a haze. I was scared. Then I did not think the baby was mine. I did nothing to 'birth' her. I did not even see her come out of me. I could not hold her for over an hour. Everyone else did but me."

Theresa, traumatic scheduled cesarean

"The overwhelming source of the trauma, for me, was the fact that I was alone in the operating room, physically strapped down and unable to move – and telling them as best I could that I was not, in fact, numb. They doubted me and kept telling me I was feeling pressure, not pain. I cannot tell you how unbelievably violated I felt at that time – a room full of strangers, me physically restrained, completely exposed, no one there who appeared familiar, and no one appearing to listen to me."

Amanda, failed anesthesia during traumatic cesarean

Traumatic birth, like other traumatic events, is a subjective experience (American Psychiatric Association, 1994; Beck, 2004a). The subjectivity of trauma explains why a woman may be traumatized by a birth that seems routine to her health care providers. Applying the diagnostic criteria elaborated in the DSM-IV (American Psychiatric Association, 1994), birth may be traumatic when a mother experiences an actual or perceived threat to her or her baby's life, serious injury to herself or her baby, threat to her or her baby's physical integrity, or her baby's death. Serious maternal injuries include episiotomy and cesarean section. Serious infant injuries include those resulting from vacuum extraction or the use of forceps. A mother may experience instrumental and surgical procedures, pelvic examinations, and external version as a threat to her or her baby's physical integrity. If a mother's response to such injuries and threats is that of intense fear, helplessness, and/or horror, then birth has been traumatic for her.

Applying DSM-IV diagnostic criteria again (American Psychiatric Association, 1994), characteristic symptoms of traumatic childbirth include persistently re-experiencing the birth, persistently avoiding stimuli associated with the birth (e.g., avoiding the health care providers involved in the birth, avoiding interaction with the baby), numbing of general responsiveness (e.g., an absence of feelings of attachment to or love for the baby), and persistent symptoms of increased arousal (e.g., insomnia, anxiety for the baby). If symptoms last more than one month and cause significant distress and impairment of functioning, the mother may meet the criteria for posttraumatic stress disorder (PTSD). If symptoms occur within four weeks of the birth and last two days to four weeks, the mother may meet the criteria for acute stress disorder (ASD).

After childbirth trauma, depression may be comorbid with PTSD or ASD or may occur alone. Depression shares several symptoms with traumatic stress disorders, including diminished interest in normal activities, irritability and anger, disturbed sleep, difficulty concentrating, and thoughts of death (American Psychiatric Association, 1994). Depression also involves symptoms of persistent sadness, disturbances in appetite and weight, psychomotor retardation or agitation, fatigue or loss of energy, and feelings of excessive guilt or worthlessness.

Mothers may arrive at birth with pre-existing characteristics and a history of experiences that increase their risk of traumatic childbirth. These maternal-related risk factors include expectation of severe labor pain; personality traits of neuroticism and anxiety; a history of psychiatric disorders such as PTSD and depression; and a history of traumatic events such as domestic violence, sexual abuse, and sexual assault (American Psychiatric Association, 1994; Bailham and Joseph, 2003; Chung *et al.*, 2001; Cohen *et al.*, 2004; Czarnocka and Slade, 2000; Dannenbring *et al.*, 1997; Issokson, 2003; Johnstone *et al.*, 2001; Kendall-Tackett, 2005a; Olde *et al.*, 2006; Seng *et al.*, 2001; Simkin and Klaus, 2004). Such risk factors are staggeringly common: approximately 22 percent of women have been sexually abused in childhood; one in six women have experienced an attempted or completed rape during their lifetimes; 20 percent to 25 percent of college women have experienced an attempted or completed rape in their lifetimes; 25 percent to 35 percent of women have been physically or sexually assaulted by an intimate partner; 13 per 1000 women in the general population have PTSD; 25 percent of women experience depression in their lifetimes; and one in 20 women experiences antenatal depression (American Psychiatric Association, 1994; Basile, 2005; Campbell and Kendall-Tackett, 2005; Helzer *et al.*, 1987; Marcus *et al.*, 2003). A significant number of women are at risk of experiencing traumatic childbirth even before labor begins.

Identifiable characteristics of labor and birth experiences also increase the risk of childbirth trauma. These birth-related risk factors include severe pain; feelings of loss of control; a birth experience that is more negative than expected; negative emotions and intrapartum dissociation; unsafe intrapartum care; inadequate emotional support from health care providers and other labor companions; long, difficult or complicated labor; negative birth outcomes, such as prematurity, pregnancy loss, and stillbirth; health care providers and family members valuing birth outcome more than birth experience; and instrumental and operative procedures, particularly emergency cesareans (Adewuya *et al.*, 2006; Ayers and Pickering, 2001; Bailham and

Joseph, 2003; Beck, 2004a, 2004b; Kendall-Tackett, 2005a, 2005b; Creedy *et al.*, 2000; Czarnocka and Slade, 2000; Olde *et al.*, 2005, 2006; Rowe-Murray and Fisher, 2001; Soet *et al.*, 2003; Turton *et al.*, 2001).

Cesarean rates are high and rising around the world. In the United States, cesarean rates have never been higher: 23.6 percent for low-risk women having a first birth and 88.7 percent for low-risk women who have had a previous cesarean (Menacker, 2005). Cesarean rates in other areas of the world are also rising: greater than 40 percent in Argentina, Brazil, and Paraguay and greater than 50 percent in Chile, Columbia, and Mexico (Kroeger and Smith, 2004). The World Health Organization (WHO) estimates that no more than 10 percent to 15 percent of all births, including those at high-risk referral facilities, should result in c-sections (WHO, 1985). Therefore, a significant proportion of cesareans in the U.S. and other countries are medically unnecessary and may cause iatrogenic trauma.

THE PREVALENCE OF CHILDBIRTH TRAUMA

"I asked the anesthesiologist what would have happened to me in the olden days and he said the mother would have died. And that's exactly what I thought when it got so scary during the surgery. That I just might die, and my baby just might die, and that I had to let go and be OK with that."

Kelly, traumatic emergency cesarean after a long labor and failed forceps delivery

"I delivered her surgically, with the on-call OB who made the experience even more traumatic with her attitude. Same for the nursing staff. . . . I felt alone and without support while in the hospital."

Maria, traumatic emergency cesarean

The prevalence of traumatic childbirth and its psychological sequelae has only recently begun to be studied. A study of sex differences in the development of PTSD in the general population showed prevalence rates of 5 per 1000 among men and 13 per 1000 among women (Helzer et al., 1987). Resnick and colleagues' (1993) study confirmed that more women than men experience PTSD. The most common type of event triggering PTSD in men is combat exposure, and in women, physical attack (e.g., rape, aggravated assault) and threats (Davidson et al., 1991; Helzer et al., 1987; Resnick et al., 1993). Childbearing women surely include a small percentage of women who are experiencing PTSD even before labor and birth begin (Reynolds, 1997).

Up to one-third of childbearing women report a traumatic birth experience and subsequent symptoms of traumatic stress (Creedy et al., 2000; Czarnocka and Slade, 2000; Declercq et al., 2008; Gamble et al., 2005; Olde et al., 2006; Soet et al., 2003). In a review by Beck (2004a), the reported prevalence of posttraumatic stress disorder following birth was found to be between 1.5 percent and 5.6 percent. If women with pre-existing risk factors for traumatic childbirth (e.g., a history of PTSD or depression) had been included in the study, these percentages would likely be significantly higher (Ayers and Pickering, 2001; Kendall-Tackett, 2005a, 2005b). In a U.S. study based on a representative national sample of 1573 new mothers, 18 percent appeared to be experiencing some PTSD symptoms, and 9 percent appeared to meet diagnostic criteria for PTSD; mothers whose babies had died – and who are inherently at risk for traumatic stress reactions – were excluded from the study (Declercq et al., 2008).

Additional factors may contribute to the underestimation of the actual prevalence of traumatic birth and resulting stress disorders. First, health care providers who routinely conduct cesareans may be unlikely to routinely evaluate new mothers for iatrogenic trauma (Madsen, 1994). Second, social desirability, the tendency to present oneself positively, can result in the reduction of reports of PTSD (Wagner et al., 1998). While this phenomenon has not yet been studied in new mothers, its impact is suggested by the frequency with which women conceal their depression due to feelings of shame, embarrassment, failure, fear of judgment, and fear that they might jeopardize their custody of the baby (Beck, 1996; Beck and Gable, 2001; Sichel *et al.*, 1993). Up to 88 percent of women with postpartum depression (PPD) are not identified because mothers are not reporting their symptoms (MacLennan *et al.*, 1996; Whitton *et al.*, 1996) and/or because health care providers are not screening for it (Beck, 1996; Beck and Gable, 2001; Cooper and Murray, 1998; Hearn *et al.*, 1998; Whitton *et al.*, 1996). Women traumatized in birth are often encouraged to value a positive birth outcome more than a negative birth experience and to focus on the future, not the past (Beck, 2004a; Good Mojab, 2000; Wolf, 2003). Such social pressures are likely to contribute to an underestimation of the actual rates of childbirth trauma and its psychological sequelae.

THE IMPACT OF TRAUMATIC CHILDBIRTH

"I was majorly depressed. I felt that if it wasn't for my child, I could kill myself. At that point I sought counseling. I cried endlessly about things. It was harder to get over because my surgical scar wouldn't heal, and when it did heal, it stayed 'disfigured.' I had no energy. It took me months to stop sleeping most of the day, to get out, to do housework. I cried when I drove, and had dreams about being coerced into a cesarean surgery all over again."

Maria, traumatic emergency cesarean

"Whenever I woke, I ate and pumped but otherwise was just checked out. After having the c-section, I felt like we were in crisis mode, but with the infection it seemed even worse and that it would never end. . . . Now nine weeks later I am struggling with postpartum depression that I think started somewhere during the birth process when I had to let go of so much."

Kelly, traumatic emergency cesarean after a long labor and failed forceps delivery

Symptoms of depression, anxiety, grief, and stress after a traumatic birth have been reported in the literature and observed clinically (e.g., Beck, 2004a, 2004b; Beck and Driscoll, 2006; Declercq et al., 2008; Fisher et al., 1997; Issokson, 2003; Kendall-Tackett, 2005a, 2005b; Murphy et al., 2003; Reynolds, 1997; Rowe-Murray and Fisher, 2001; Ryding, 1991, 1993; Turton et al., 2001). For example, a traumatized mother may experience a severe impairment of self-worth, as well as feelings of failure and guilt. Her ability to emotionally bond and interact with her baby may be impaired. She may experience intrusive thoughts about the birth – like a tape being played over and over again. Her ability to fall and stay asleep may be seriously impaired due to hyperarousal, intrusive thoughts, and terrifying nightmares related to the birth. A mother may not remember all or part of labor and birth or she may remember it only with pain, anger, fear, or sadness. She may deeply grieve the loss of her expected birth experience. A traumatized mother may be unable to resume sexual relations or may avoid childbearing. If she does become pregnant again, she may experience the return of symptoms of traumatic stress and may choose an elective cesarean to avoid a vaginal birth or to increase a sense of control over her upcoming labor and birth experience. When a woman is terrified of experiencing a traumatic birth again, she may even choose the early termination of a subsequent pregnancy.

The impact of maternal traumatic stress on infant well-being and development has not yet been studied. However, research on PPD suggests that it is likely to be negative. Extensive research shows that PPD increases the risk of many emotional, behavioral, and developmental problems in infancy and childhood and the risk of depression in adulthood (Beck and Driscoll, 2006; Kendall-Tackett, 2005b). While not examining traumatic stress due to childbirth, Rowe-Murray and Fisher's (2001) study found that instrumental and surgical births (risk factors for childbirth trauma) negatively impacted postnatal maternal-infant contact with persistent concomitant negative maternal emotional outcomes, including a greater risk of maternal depression.

THE IMPACT OF CHILDBIRTH TRAUMA ON BREASTFEEDING

"I desired exclusive breastfeeding from the minute he was born. I didn't even consider that this wouldn't happen. I think the birth trauma made me both panicked and withdrawn, and I don't know how much that influenced the fact that breastfeeding didn't work out. I know it contributed to my postpartum depression, and I don't know whether the depression or the failure of breastfeeding was the chicken or the egg."

> Kelly, traumatic emergency cesarean after a long labor and failed forceps delivery

"Immediately after the birth I was confused, feeling helpless with this child, so tired. . . . I didn't realize it then, but the postpartum depression I would later get diagnosed with was beginning. I didn't want to hold him. I didn't know how to care for him. I was annoyed at him for putting me through all of that and outraged that things were so messy with the labor and birth. . . . It was like all of the odds were completely stacked against my ever being able to nurse him. . . . I still feel guilty about it to this day."

> Victoria, traumatic labor and cesarean

Clinical experience shows that depression, anxiety, sleep deprivation due to hyperarousal, avoidance of the baby, and lack of emotion toward the baby may all contribute to the undermining of breastfeeding after childbirth trauma. However, research on the impact of traumatic birth experiences on breastfeeding is in its infancy. Many questions remain as to how greatly physical as well as emotional trauma impact breastfeeding. Studies on the prevalence of traumatic stress reactions following childbirth trauma have not provided information on mothering behavior or infant feeding (e.g., Creedy *et al.*, 2000; Soet *et al.*, 2003). The results of research on the impact of cesarean on breastfeeding reflect varying study designs, confounding factors (e.g., maternal–infant separation), and the intertwined physical and psychological impact of surgical birth on a mother's ability to breastfeed. Many studies have shown that operative births are associated with delayed lactogenesis, and subsequently a delayed initiation of breastfeeding (Chen *et al.*, 1998; Dewey *et al.*, 2003; Evans *et al.*, 2003; Grajeda and Pérez-Escamilla, 2002; Leung *et al.*, 2002; Nissen *et al.*, 1996; Rowe-Murray and Fisher, 2002; Vestermark *et al.*, 1991; Wittels *et al.*, 1997). Other studies have shown that breastfeeding duration does not differ significantly between mothers who give birth surgically or vaginally (Kearney *et al.*, 1990b; Victora *et al.*, 1990). However, breastfeeding duration after emergency cesarean is shorter than after planned cesarean (Victora *et al.*, 1990).

Cesarean birth, like any other form of major surgery, requires a significant amount of time for recovery. The stress, injury, pain, analgesics, and anesthetics involved may prevent a mother from breastfeeding in a manner (e.g., early and often) that facilitates the development of an ample milk supply. Analgesics and anesthetics used during labor and birth also affect the baby born by cesarean, causing lethargy and disorientation and an impaired ability to breastfeed (see Kroeger and Smith, 2004, for a review; Righard and Alade, 1990). Maternal–infant separation, a common outcome of operative birth, negatively affects postnatal maternal–infant interaction (Rowe-Murray and Fisher, 2001) and impairs infant ability to breastfeed (Righard and Alade, 1990).

Impaired mental health, in any form, inherently leaves a mother poorly equipped to initiate breastfeeding and to cope with breastfeeding problems. Research results on the direction of the causal relationship between poor maternal mental health and breastfeeding are somewhat conflicting. However, the majority of studies indicate an inverse relationship between breastfeeding and PPD or an earlier cessation of breastfeeding when PPD (Abou-Saleh *et al.*, 1998; Cooper *et al.*, 1993; Falceto *et al.*, 2004; Fergerson *et al.*, 2002; Galler *et al.*, 1999; Green and Murray, 1994; Hannah *et al.*, 1992; Hellin and Waller, 1992;

Kearney *et al.*, 1990a; Tarkka *et al.*, 1999; Taveras *et al.*, 2003; Warner *et al.*, 1996) or anxiety (Scrimshaw *et al.*, 1987) is present. Henderson and colleagues (2003) found that an early cessation of breastfeeding was significantly associated with PPD – and that in most cases the onset of PPD preceded the breastfeeding cessation. Misri and colleagues (1997) found that depression preceded breastfeeding cessation in 83 percent of mothers. Taj and Sikander (2003) found that 36.8 percent of mothers reported that their depressive symptoms began before weaning occurred.

Breastfeeding initiation may be more vulnerable relative to its continuance once breastfeeding is well established (Falceto *et al.*, 2004; Hatton *et al.*, 2005). Adequate social support may lessen the impact of PPD on breastfeeding (Falceto *et al.*, 2004; Kendall-Tackett, 2005b). The authors of a recent study related to PPD and breastfeeding noted that, in studies which did not find an inverse relationship between breastfeeding and maternal depression, data were obtained later in the postpartum period or were combined across the entire postpartum measurement period (Hatton *et al.*, 2005). In addition, women who wean earlier than they had expected often experience feelings of sadness, loss, disappointment, inadequacy, failure in attaining the maternal role, and invalidation (Chezem *et al.*, 1997; Coreil and Murphy, 1988; Driscoll, 1992). Therefore, it should not be surprising that depressive symptoms, such as sadness, anger, and guilt (which also occur during grief [Worden, 2002]) can follow, as well as precede, breastfeeding cessation. I have worked with many mothers grieving deeply over the complete or partial loss of breastfeeding.

The means by which poor maternal mental health can impact breastfeeding appears to include the undermining of mothering behaviors and maternal–infant interactions that are supportive of breastfeeding. Difficulties in maternal–infant interactions (i.e., sensitivity to cues, response to distress, social-emotional growth fostering, cognitive growth fostering, clarity of cues, responsiveness to parent) 29 to 90 hours after birth are related to an earlier cessation of breastfeeding (Brandt *et al.*, 1998). A mother experiencing symptoms of traumatic stress would logically find it more difficult to respond sensitively to her infant's cues (e.g., feeding cues), respond to her infant's distress, and foster her infant's growth than a mother who has not been traumatized in birth. Numerous studies have shown how PPD impairs maternal expressiveness, involvement, responsiveness, sensitivity, physical contact, engagement, and supportiveness toward their infants (Albertsson-Karlgren *et al.*, 2001; Beck, 1995; Field, 1992; Righetti-Veltema *et al.*, 2002; Tronick and Weinberg, 1997). These behaviors are the very types that are associated with earlier weaning (Brandt *et al.*, 1998).

Through my research and in my counseling practice, many women have shared with me the various ways in which a traumatic birth affected their experience of breastfeeding. Some women become even more desirous of breastfeeding in an effort to have something "go right," to emotionally heal, or to overcome their emotional detachment from their baby. However, the magnitude of a mother's emotional trauma can undermine breastfeeding in spite of a strong desire. Women may struggle with an emotional detachment from their infant and the desire to avoid interacting with their infant, which can negatively impact the quality and duration of their breastfeeding experience. Their symptoms of traumatic stress and depression may leave them too overwhelmed to find solutions to breastfeeding problems following a traumatic birth experience. If they seek mental health care, breastfeeding may be undermined by recommendations to wean due to the mistaken impression that weaning is guaranteed to relieve their psychological distress or that the use of psychotropic medications always contraindicates breastfeeding. However, most medications are compatible with breastfeeding (Hale, 2006). The breastfeeding experience of traumatized mothers may be significantly shorter than they expected, increasing their symptoms of grief and exposing them and their infants to health risks due to the introduction of artificial substitutes for human milk.

"I was too consumed with my own pain to be able to bond with my child immediately. Breastfeeding was very much a practical matter the first few weeks and I think that set the tone for my entire breastfeeding experience with her."

Amanda, traumatic cesarean after failed induction

"I ruptured and immediately had a very painful, very, very scary c-section. It lives in all my nightmares. During the section, when I was screaming my head off, the doctor told me that my baby wasn't going to make it. . . . I cried a lot and suffered depression for a very long time – probably still do. I loved my baby and worried constantly about her health. I was in too much pain. I felt like a failure. My milk never came in at all. I had nothing to feed her. I couldn't hold her long enough to nurse."

Barbara, traumatic induced labor and repeat cesarean

"I wanted to breastfeed so badly. I looked forward to the bonding, and closeness. . . . the horrible shoulder pain I was having when holding her brought tears to my eyes. I would cry. She would cry. She gave up. She was hungry and I had nothing. I started pumping and feeding as soon as anything came in. But I was so tense. It was so mechanical. . . . I could not take it anymore. I could not do it. I cried because not only did they take my birth from me, but they took my ability to breastfeed and bond with my child."

Theresa, traumatic scheduled cesarean

Health care providers, friends and family may not realize how important breastfeeding can be to a mother after a traumatic birth experience. After three second-trimester miscarriages, Nanette lost a twin at 8 weeks. When her surviving baby was born, he was not expected to live for more than 24 hours due to multiple complications from an infection he contracted *in utero*.

Although he survived, Nanette was left with severe PPD and traumatic stress.

> "There were days when I felt I had nothing to live for but I knew that if I wasn't around, my baby would be given formula. Knowing that I had to be there to breastfeed my baby literally prevented me from killing myself a couple of times. I wanted to be sure that my son had that bonding experience and I knew that breastfeeding was the healthiest thing I could do for him."
>
> Nanette, traumatic prolonged vaginal birth

INFANT AND MATERNAL HEALTH RISKS OF UNDERMINING BREASTFEEDING

The undermining of breastfeeding as a possible outcome of traumatic birth warrants the attention of health care providers. Infant feeding is a major health issue. Formula feeding poses numerous and significant risks to children in both developed and developing countries, including greater risk of illness, disease, allergic manifestations, hospitalization, and death in infancy; learning and cognitive deficiencies in children aged 1 through 18 years of age; and, among mothers who formula feed, higher rates of disease, including breast and ovarian cancer, anemia, and osteoporosis (e.g., American Academy of Pediatrics, 2005; Chen and Rogan, 2004; Lawrence, 1997, 2001; Walker, 1992, 1993, 1998, 2004, 2005).

Mothers traumatized in birth have fewer resources available to cope with the needs of a newborn and any challenges – including those related to breastfeeding – that may arise postpartum. Breastfeeding problems may quickly result in the introduction of artificial substitutes for human milk. Many health care providers are not familiar with the large evidence base demonstrating the risks involved in doing so. Before 6 months of age, even a single feeding of infant formula is not a benign intervention (American Academy of Pediatrics, 2005; Walker, 1992, 1993, 1998, 2004, 2005). The negative impact of the introduction of feeding an infant even a small amount of formula is immediately evidenced by disturbances in the state and behavior of the infant gut (Walker, 2005). Infants born by cesarean, born prematurely, requiring intensive care, and/or separated from their mothers – infants born to the very mothers that are more likely to have experienced intrapartum trauma – are at greatest risk of colonization by harmful microbes because they have not had the opportunity for colonization by their mothers' bacteria through vaginal birth and/or because their primary exposure is to environmental bacteria rather than their mothers'. The introduction of breastmilk substitutes even further impairs the state and behavior of the gut of these already vulnerable infants and further increases their risk of disease.

In recognition of the risks of formula feeding, the American Academy of Pediatrics (2005) recommends that breastfeeding continue for at least one year. Breastfeeding a child for at least two years is recommended by the United Nations Children's Fund (UNICEF) and WHO (UNICEF, 2002). The AAP and WHO both recommend exclusive breastfeeding during the first six months of life, with appropriate table foods and beverages gradually introduced after about 6 months of age. While such recommendations run counter to widespread cultural norms of early weaning and the use of artificial substitutes for human milk, they support biologically normal patterns of health and development among human beings.

IMPLICATIONS FOR PRACTICE

The prevention and reduction of the negative impact of traumatic birth on mothers and infants can only be accomplished through the coordinated efforts of a diverse group of health care providers – antenatally, intrapartum, and postpartum. Good communication and "power sharing" between women and their health care providers is essential for women to be able to more actively participate in their childbearing experience, lessening their risk of feeling a loss of control during labor and birth, and decreasing their risk of a traumatic birth experience (for models of partnership in health care see Leff and Walizer, 1992; Rosenburg, 2003; Simkin and Klaus, 2004).

Prenatal strategies for the prevention and reduction of the risk and severity of childbirth trauma include: (1) screening for maternal-related risk factors for childbirth trauma; (2) childbirth classes that offer women the opportunity to learn how such factors can increase their risk of traumatic childbirth; (3) assessing the woman's emotional response to physical examinations during pregnancy and her concerns about the upcoming labor and birth; and (4) referral of at-risk women to mental health care providers who specialize in helping women to emotionally prepare for birth (Goldbeck-Wood, 1996; Reynolds, 1997; Ryding, 1991, 1993; Simkin and Klaus, 2004).

Strategies for reducing the risk and severity of trauma during labor and birth include: (1) creating an environment in which positive birth experiences are possible; for example, by implementing the ten steps of the Mother-friendly Childbirth Initiative (CIMS, 1996; Reynolds, 1997; Simkin and Klaus, 2004); and (2) the evidence-based management of maternal acute traumatic stress, for example, by reducing exposure to traumatizing sensory input, avoiding maternal-infant separation, screening for maternal- and birth-related risk factors for traumatic birth, screening for symptoms of traumatic stress, and responding to emergent maternal psychological needs (Lerner and Shelton, 2005).

Postpartum strategies for responding to and reducing the severity and duration of symptoms of childbirth trauma include: (1) screening for maternal- and birth-related risk factors for trauma; (2) ongoing screening for traumatic stress, depression, and grief; (3) postpartum birth debriefing, including asking the mother about her experience and answering any questions she has (Gamble et al., 2005); (4) implementation of the "ten steps to successful breastfeeding" of the Baby Friendly Hospital Initiative (UNICEF/WHO, 2006); (5) implementation of "kangaroo care" (skin-to-skin care and breastfeeding of the neonate)

(Anderson *et al.*, 2004); (6) providing extra breastfeeding information and support; (7) referral to an International Board Certified Lactation Consultant (IBCLC) experienced with breastfeeding management and support after childbirth trauma; (8) referral to support groups, such as chapter meetings of the International Cesarean Awareness Network (www.ican-online.org), and therapy groups for recovery from childbirth trauma (Sorenson, 2003); (9) referral to mental health professionals specializing in recovery from childbirth trauma and lactational psychology (Good Mojab, 2006); (10) providing breastfeeding mothers with evidence-based information about the use of psychotropic medications (Hale, 2006); and (11) providing mothers with information about contraception if they wish to avoid pregnancy (Reynolds, 1997).

SUMMARY

A significant number of women are at risk of experiencing a psychologically traumatic labor and birth. Traumatic stress can impair maternal mental health and behavior, including breastfeeding. When breastfeeding is undermined, infants are exposed to artificial substitutes for human milk, increasing numerous, significant health risks for both mother and child. Health care providers can do much to identify mothers at risk for traumatic birth experiences, prevent iatrogenic trauma during labor and birth, and identify and refer traumatized mothers to mental health care providers and IBCLCs specializing in working with mothers traumatized during birth. Prevention of the impairment of maternal and infant health through the undermining of breastfeeding after childbirth trauma requires a comprehensive approach to the care of childbearing women.

REFERENCES

Abou-Saleh, M., Ghubash, R., Karim, L., Krymski, M., and Bhai, I. (1998). Hormonal aspects of postpartum depression. *Psychoneuroendocrinology*, *23*(5), 465–475.

Adewuya, A., Ologun, Y., and Ibigbami, O. (2006). Post-traumatic stress disorder after childbirth in Nigerian women: Prevalence and risk factors. *British Journal of Obstetrics and Gynaecology, 113*(3), 284–288.

Albertsson-Karlgren, U., Graff, M., and Nettelbladt, P. (2001). Mental disease postpartum and parent-infant interaction: Evaluation of videotaped sessions. *Child Abuse Review, 10*(1), 5–17.

American Academy of Pediatrics (2005). Breastfeeding and the use of human milk (RE9729). *Pediatrics, 115*(2), 496–506.

American Psychiatric Association (1994). *Diagnostic and statistical manual of mental disorders (fourth edition)*. Washington, DC: American Psychiatric Association.

Anderson, G., Moore, E., Hepworth, J., and Bergman, N. (2004). Early skin-to-skin contact for mothers and their healthy newborn infants (Cochrane Review). In *The Cochrane Library*, Issue 2. Chichester, UK: John Wiley & Sons.

Ayers, S., and Pickering, A. (2001). Do women get posttraumatic stress disorder as a result of childbirth? A prospective study of incidence. *Birth, 28*, 111–118.

Bailham, D., and Joseph, S. (2003). Post-traumatic stress following childbirth: A review of the emerging literature and directions for research and practice. *Psychology, Health and Medicine, 8*(2), 159–168.

Basile, K. (2005). Sexual violence in the lives of girls and women. In K. Kendall-Tackett (ed.), *Handbook of women, stress, and trauma* (pp. 101–122). New York: Brunner-Routledge.

Beck, C. (1995). The effects of postpartum depression on maternal-infant interaction: A meta-analysis. *Nursing Research, 44*, 298–304.

Beck, C. (1996). A meta-analysis of predictors of postpartum depression. *Nursing Research, 45*(5), 297–303.

Beck, C. (2004a). Birth trauma: In the eye of the beholder. *Nursing Research, 53*(1), 28–35.

Beck, C. (2004b). Post-traumatic stress disorder due to childbirth: The aftermath. *Nursing Research, 53*, 216–224.

Beck, C., and Driscoll, J.W. (2006). *Postpartum mood disorders*. Sudbury, MA: Jones & Bartlett.

Beck, C., and Gable, R. (2001). Further validation of the Postpartum Depression Screening Scale. *Nursing Research, 50*, 155–164.

Brandt, K., Andrews, C., and Kvale, J. (1998). Mother–infant interaction and breastfeeding outcome 6 weeks after birth. *Journal of Obstetric, Gynecologic, and Neonatal Nursing, 27*(2), 169–174.

Campbell, J., and Kendall-Tackett, K. (2005). Intimate partner violence: Implications for women's physical and mental health. In K. Kendall-Tackett (ed.), *Handbook of women, stress, and trauma* (pp. 123–140). New York: Brunner-Routledge.

Chen, A., and Rogan, W. (2004). Breastfeeding and the risk of postneonatal death in the United States. *Pediatrics, 113*(5), e435–439.

Chen, D., Nommsen-Rivers, L., Dewey, K., and Lonnerdal, B. (1998). Stress during labor and delivery and early lactation performance. *The American Journal of Clinical Nutrition, 68*(2), 334–344.

Chezem, J., Montgomery, P., and Fortman, T. (1997). Maternal feelings after cessation of breastfeeding: Influence of factors related to employment and duration. *The Journal of Perinatal and Neonatal Nursing, 11*(2), 61–70.

Chung, T., Lau, T., Yip, A., Chiu, H., and Lee, D. (2001). Antepartum depressive symptomatology is associated with adverse obstetric and neonatal outcomes. *Psychosomatic Medicine, 63*, 830–834.

Coalition for Improving Maternity Services (CIMS) (1996). Mother-friendly childbirth initiative. www.motherfriendly.org/mfci.

Cohen, M., Ansara, D., Schei, B., Stuckless, N., and Stewart, D. (2004). Posttraumatic stress disorder after pregnancy, labor, and delivery. *Journal of Women's Health, 13*(3), 315–324.

Cooper, P., and Murray, L. (1998). Postnatal depression. *British Medical Journal, 316*, 1884–1886.

Cooper, P., Murray, L., and Stein, A. (1993). Psychosocial factors associated with the early termination of breast-feeding. *Journal of Psychiatric Research, 37*, 171–176.

Coreil, J., and Murphy, E. (1988). Maternal commitment, lactation practices, and breastfeeding duration. *Journal of Obstetric, Gynecologic, and Neonatal Nursing, 17*, 273–278.

Creedy, D., Shochet, I., and Horsfall, J. (2000). Childbirth and the development of acute trauma symptoms: Incidence and contributing factors. *Birth, 27*(2), 104–111.

Czarnocka, J., and Slade, P. (2000). Prevalence and predictors of post-traumatic stress symptoms following childbirth. *The British Journal of Clinical Psychology, 39*, 35–51.

Dannenbring, D., Stevens, M., and House, A. (1997). Predictors of childbirth pain and maternal satisfaction. *Journal of Behavioral Medicine, 20*(2), 127–142.

Davidson, J., Hughes, D., Blazer, D., and George, L. (1991). Post-traumatic stress disorders in the community: Epidemiological study. *Psychological Medicine, 21*(3), 713–721.

Declercq, E., Sakala, C., Corry, M., and Applebaum, S. (2008). *New Mothers Speak Out: National Survey Results Highlight Women's Postpartum Experiences*. New York: Childbirth Connection.

Dewey, K., Nommsen-Rivers, L., Heinig, J., and Cohen, R. (2003). Risk factors for suboptimal infant breastfeeding behavior, delayed onset of lactation, and excess neonatal weight loss. *Pediatrics, 112*(3), 607–619.

Driscoll, J. (1992). Breastfeeding success and failure: Implications for nurses. In *NAACOG clinical issues in perinatal and women's health nursing* (pp. 565–569). Philadelphia, PA: Lippincott.

Evans, K., Evans, R., Royal, R., Esterman, A., and James, S. (2003). Effect of caesarean section on breast milk transfer to the normal term newborn over the first week of life. *Archives of Disease in Childhood. Fetal and Neonatal Edition, 88*(5), F380–382.

Falceto, O., Giugliani, E., and Fernandes, C. (2004). Influence of parental mental health on early termination of breast-feeding: A case-control study. *Journal of the American Board of Family Practice, 17*(3), 173–183.

Fergerson, S., Jamieson, D., and Lindsay, M. (2002). Diagnosing postpartum depression: Can we do better? *American Journal of Obstetrics and Gynecology, 186*(5), 899–902.

Field, T. (1992). Infants of depressed mothers. *Development and Psychopathology, 4*, 49–66.

Fisher, J., Astbury, J., and Smith, A. (1997). Adverse psychological impact of operative obstetric interventions: A prospective longitudinal study. *Australian and New Zealand Journal of Psychiatry, 31*, 728–738.

Galler, J., Harrison, R., Biggs, M., Ramsey, F., and Forde, V. (1999). Maternal moods predict breastfeeding in Barbados. *Journal of Developmental and Behavioral Pediatrics, 20*, 80–87.

Gamble, J., Creedy, D., Moyle, W., Webster, J., McAllister, M., and Dickson, P. (2005). Effectiveness of a counseling intervention after a traumatic childbirth: A randomized controlled trial. *Birth, 32*(1), 11–19.

Goldbeck-Wood, S. (1996). PTSD may follow childbirth. *British Medical Journal, 313,* 774.

Good Mojab, C. (2000). The cultural art of breastfeeding. *Leaven, 36*(5), 87–91.

Good Mojab, C. (2006). Regarding the emerging field of lactational psychology. *Journal of Human Lactation, 22*(1), 13–14.

Grajeda, R., and Pérez-Escamilla, R. (2002). Stress during labor and delivery is associated with delayed onset of lactation among urban Guatemalan women. *Journal of Nutrition, 132*(10), 3055–3060.

Green, J., and Murray, D. (1994). The use of the Edinburgh Postnatal Depression Scale in research to explore the relationship between antenatal and postnatal dysphoria. In J. Cox and J. Holden (eds), *Perinatal psychiatry: Use and misuse of the Edinburgh Postnatal Depression Scale* (pp. 180–198). London: Gaskell.

Hale, T. (2006). *Medications and mothers' milk: A manual of lactational pharmacology.* Amarillo, TX: Hale Publishing.

Hannah, P., Adams, D., Lee, A., Glover, V., and Sandler, M. (1992). Links between early post-partum mood and postnatal depression. *British Journal of Psychiatry, 160,* 777–780.

Hatton, D., Harrison-Hohner, J., Coste, S., Dorato, V., Curet, L., and McCarron, D. (2005). Symptoms of postpartum depression and breastfeeding. *Journal of Human Lactation, 21*(4), 444–449.

Hearn, G., Iliff, A., Jones I., Kirby, A., Ormiston, P., Parr, P., *et al.* (1998). Postnatal depression in the community. *British Journal of General Practice, 48,* 1064–1066.

Hellin, K., and Waller, G. (1992). Mothers' mood and infant feeding: Prediction of problems and practices. *Journal of Reproductive and Infant Psychology, 10,* 39–51.

Helzer, J., Robins, L., and McEvoy, L. (1987). Post traumatic stress disorder in the general population: Findings of the epidemiologic catchment area survey. *New England Journal of Medicine, 317,* 1630–1634.

Henderson, J., Evans, S., Straton, J., Priest, S., and Hagan, R (2003). Impact of postnatal depression on breastfeeding duration. *Birth, 30*(3), 175–180.

Issokson, D. (2003). Effects of childhood abuse on childbearing and perinatal health. In K. Kendall-Tackett (ed.), *Health consequences of abuse in the family: A clinical guide for evidence-based practice* (pp. 197–214). Washington, DC: American Psychological Association.

Johnstone, S., Boyce, P., Hickey, A., Morris-Yates, A., and Harris, M. (2001). Obstetric risk factors for postnatal depression in urban and rural community samples. *Australian and New Zealand Journal of Psychiatry, 35*(1), 69–74.

Kearney, M., Cronenwett, L., and Barrett, J. (1990a). Breastfeeding problems in the first week postpartum. *Nursing Research, 39*, 90–95.

Kearney, M., Cronenwett, L., and Reinhardt, R. (1990b). Cesarean delivery and breastfeeding outcomes. *Birth, 17*(2), 97–103.

Kendall-Tackett, K. (2005a). Trauma associated with perinatal events: Birth experience, prematurity, and childbearing loss. In K. Kendall-Tackett (ed.), *Handbook of women, stress, and trauma* (pp. 53–74). New York: Brunner-Routledge.

Kendall-Tackett, K. (2005b). *Depression in new mothers: Causes, consequences, and treatment alternatives*. Binghamton, NY: The Haworth Press.

Kroeger, M., and Smith, L. (2004). *Impact of birthing practices on breastfeeding: Protecting the mother and baby continuum*. Sudbury, MA: Jones & Bartlett.

Lawrence, R. (1997). National Association of Pediatric Nurse Practitioners. Position statement on breastfeeding. *Journal of Pediatric Health Care, 15*, 22A.

Lawrence, R. (2001). *A review of the medical benefits and contraindications to breastfeeding in the United States*, Arlington, VA: National Center for Education in Maternal and Child Health.

Leff, P., and Walizer, E. (1992). *Building the healing partnership: Parents, professionals, and children with chronic illnesses and disabilities*. Brookline, MA: Brookline Books.

Lerner, M. and Shelton, R. (2005). *Comprehensive acute traumatic stress management: A traumatic stress response protocol for all caregivers*. New York: The American Academy of Experts in Traumatic Stress.

Leung, G., Lam, T., and Ho, L. (2002). Breast-feeding and its relation to smoking and mode of delivery. *Obstetrics and Gynecology, 99*, 785–794.

MacLennan, A., Wilson, D., and Taylor, A. (1996). The self-reported prevalence of postnatal depression. *Australian and New Zealand Journal of Obstetric and Gynecology, 36*, 313.

Madsen, L. (1994). *Rebounding from childbirth: Toward emotional recovery*. Westport, CT: Bergin & Garvey.

Marcus, S., Flynn, H., Blow, F., and Barry, K. (2003). Depressive symptoms among pregnant women screened in obstetric settings. *Journal of Women's Health, 12*(4), 373–380.

Menacker, F. (2005). Trends in cesarean rates for first births and repeat cesarean rates for low-risk women: United States 1990–2003. CDC *National Vital Statistics Report, 54*(4), 1–12.

Misri, S., Sinclair, D., and Kuan, A. (1997). Breast-feeding and postpartum depression: Is there a relationship? *Canadian Journal of Psychiatry, 42*, 1061–1065.

Murphy, D., Pope. C., Frost, J., and Liebling, R. (2003). Women's views on the impact of operative delivery in the second stage of labour: Qualitative interview study. *British Medical Journal, 327*, 1132–1136.

Nissen, E., Uvnas-Moberg, K., Svensson, K., Stock, S., Widstrom, A., and Winberg, J. (1996). Different patterns of oxytocin, prolactin but not cortisol release during breastfeeding in women delivered by Cesarean section or by the vaginal route. *Early Human Development, 45*(1–2), 103–118.

Olde, E., van der Hart, O., Kleber, R., van Son, M., Wijnen, H., and Pop, V. (2005). Peritraumatic dissociation and emotions as predictors of PTSD symptoms following childbirth. *Journal of Trauma and Dissociation, 6*(3), 125–142.

Olde, E., van der Hart, O., Kleber, R., and Van Son, M. (2006). Posttraumatic stress following childbirth: A review. *Clinical Psychology Review, 26*(1), 1–16.

Resnick, H., Kilpatrick, D., Dansky, B., Saunders, B., and Best, C. (1993). Prevalence of civilian trauma and posttraumatic stress disorder in a representative national sample of women. *Journal of Consulting and Clinical Psychology, 61*(6), 984–991.

Reynolds, J. (1997). Post-traumatic stress disorder after childbirth: The phenomenon of traumatic birth. *Canadian Medical Association Journal, 156*(6), 831–835.

Righard, L., and Alade, M. (1990). Effect of delivery room routines on success of first breast-feed. *Lancet, 336*(8723), 1105–1107.

Righetti-Veltema, M., Conne-Perreard, E., Bousquet, A., and Manzano, J. (2002). Postpartum depression and mother–infant relationship at 3 months old. *Journal of Affective Disorders, 70*, 291–306.

Rosenburg, M. (2003). *Nonviolent communication: A language of life.* Encinitas, CA: PuddleDancer Press.

Rowe-Murray, H., and Fisher, J. (2001). Operative intervention in delivery is associated with compromised early mother–infant interaction. *British Journal of Obstetrics and Gynaecology, 108*(10), 1068–1075.

Rowe-Murray, H., and Fisher, J. (2002). Baby friendly hospital practices: Cesarean section is a persistent barrier to early initiation of breastfeeding. *Birth, 29*(2), 124–131.

Ryding, E. (1991). Psychosocial indications for cesarean section: A retrospective study of 43 cases. *Acta Obstetricia et Gynecologica Scandinavica, 70*, 47–49.

Ryding, E. (1993). Investigation of 33 women who demanded a cesarean section for personal reasons. *Acta Obstetricia et Gynecologica Scandinavica, 72*, 280–285.

Scrimshaw, S., Engle, P., Arnold, L., and Haynes, K. (1987). Factors affecting breastfeeding among women of Mexican origin or descent in Los Angeles. *American Journal of Public Health, 77*, 467–470.

Seng, J., Oakley, D., Sampselle, C., Killion, C., Graham-Bermann, S., and Liberzon, I. (2001). Posttraumatic stress disorder and pregnancy complications. *Obstetrics and Gynecology, 97*, 17–22.

Shealy, K., Li, R., Benton-Davis, S., and Grummer-Strawn, L.M. (2005). *The CDC guide to breastfeeding interventions.* Atlanta, GA: US Department of Health and Human Services, Centers for Disease Control and Prevention.

Sichel, D., Cohen, L., Dimmock, J., and Rosenbaum, J. (1993). Postpartum obsessive compulsive disorder: A case series. *Journal of Clinical Psychiatry, 54*, 156–159.

Simkin, P., and Klaus, P. (2004). *When survivors give birth: Understanding and healing the effects of early sexual abuse on childbearing women.* Seattle, WA: Classic Day Publishing.

Soet, J., Brack, G., and Dilorio, C. (2003). Prevalence and predictors of women's experience of psychological trauma during childbirth. *Birth, 30*(1), 36–48.

Sorenson, D. (2003). Healing traumatizing provider interactions among women through short-term group therapy. *Archives of Psychiatric Nursing, 17*(6), 259–269.

Taj, R., and Sikander, K. (2003). Effects of maternal depression on breast-feeding. *Journal of the Pakistan Medical Association, 53*(1), 8–11.

Tarkka, M., Paunonen, M., and Laippala, P. (1999). Factors related to successful breast feeding by first-time mothers when the child is 3 months old. *Journal of Advanced Nursing, 29*, 113–118.

Taveras, E., Capra, A., Braveman, P., Jensvold, N., Escobar, G., and Lieu, T. (2003). Clinician support and psychosocial risk factors associated with breastfeeding discontinuation. *Pediatrics, 112*, 108–115.

Tronick, E., and Weinberg, M. (1997). Depressed mothers and infants: Failure to form dyadic states of consciousness. In L. Murray and P. Cooper (eds), *Postpartum depression and child development* (pp. 54–81). New York: Guilford Press.

Turton, P., Hughes, P., Evans, C., and Fainman, D. (2001). Incidence, correlates and predictors of post-traumatic stress disorder in the pregnancy after stillbirth. *British Journal of Psychiatry, 178*, 556–560.

UNICEF (2002). *Facts for life 2002*. New York: Author.

UNICEF/WHO (2006). *Baby Friendly Hospital Initiative, revised, updated and expanded for integrated care, Section 1, Background and implementation, Preliminary version*. New York: Author.

Vestermark, V., Hogdall, C., Birch, M., Plenov, G., and Toftager-Larsen, K. (1991). Influence of the mode of delivery on initiation of breast-feeding. *European Journal of Obstetrics, Gynecology, and Reproductive Biology, 38*(1), 33–38.

Victora, C., Huttly, S., Barros, F., and Vaughan, J. (1990). Cesarean section and duration of breast feeding among Brazilians. *Archives of Disease in Childhood, 65*(6), 632–634.

Wagner, D., Heinrichs, M., and Ehlert, U. (1998). Prevalence of symptoms of posttraumatic stress disorder in German professional firefighters. *The American Journal of Psychiatry, 155*(12), 1727–1732.

Walker, M. (1992). *Summary of the hazards of infant formula*. Raleigh, NC: International Lactation Consultant Association.

Walker, M. (1993). A fresh look at the risk of artificial infant feeding. *Journal of Human Lactation, 9*(2), 97–107.

Walker, M. (1998). *Summary of the hazards of infant formula: Part 2*. Raleigh, NC: International Lactation Consultant Association.

Walker, M. (2004). *Summary of the hazards of infant formula: Monograph 3*. Raleigh, NC: International Lactation Consultant Association.

Walker, M. (2005). *Supplementation of the breastfed baby: "Just one bottle won't hurt" – or will it?* (revised edn). Weston, MA: Lactation Associates.

Warner, R., Appleby, L., Whitton, A., and Faragher, B. (1996). Demographic and obstetric risk factors for postnatal psychiatric morbidity. *The British Journal of Psychiatry, 168*(5), 607–611.

Whitton, A., Warner, R., and Appleby, L. (1996). The pathway to care in post-natal depression: Women's attitudes to post-natal depression and its treatment. *The British Journal of General Practice, 46*, 427–428.

WHO (1985). Appropriate technology for birth. *Lancet, 2*, 436–437.

Wittels, B., Glosten, B., Faure, E., Moawad, A., Ismail, M., Hibbard, J., *et al.* (1997). Postcesarean analgesia with both epidural morphine and intravenous patient-controlled analgesia: Neurobehavioral outcomes among nursing neonates. *Anesthesia and Analgesia, 85*(3), 600–606.

Wolf, N. (2003). *Misconceptions: Truth, lies, and the unexpected on the journey to motherhood*. New York: Bantam Doubleday Dell Publishing Group.

Worden, J. (2002). *Grief counseling and grief therapy: A handbook for the mental health practitioner*. New York: Springer Publishing.

The complexity of links between physical health and trauma

The role of gender

Victoria L. Banyard

A GROWING BODY of empirical research documents important links between trauma exposure and physical health problems (e.g., Kendall-Tackett, 2004). This research has done much to improve interventions for trauma survivors; yet, to date, much of the research in this area has focused on women and women's health. Several recent studies highlight the need to consider applying a gender lens to this literature to set an agenda for future research and practice. The aim of this chapter is to review research on trauma and primary care using such a gender lens. I provide recommendations for research and practice that stem from complex definitions of gender and an appreciation of both gender similarity and difference among trauma survivors.

WHY ATTEND TO TRAUMA IN PRIMARY CARE?

Accumulated empirical research on trauma and physical health highlights the ways in which this is a critical topic for primary care. Most importantly, many studies show strong links between the experience of trauma and physical health outcomes including more negative evaluations of overall health, increases in risky health behaviors, and increased risk for life-threatening diseases with exposure to traumatic events (e.g., Arias, 2004; Edwards *et al.*, 2004; Felitti *et al.*, 1998; Lang *et al.*, 2003; Nicolaidis *et al.*, 2004; Plichta and Falik, 2001; Rodgers *et al.*, 2004; Ullman and Breklin, 2003; Ullman and Siegel, 1996). Given this potential role of trauma in the etiology of medical conditions and physical health symptoms practitioners have been encouraged to include screening for a range of traumatic events when obtaining a medical history (e.g., Edwards *et al.*, 2004).

PREVENTION AND INTERVENTION IN PRIMARY CARE
Medical settings, including primary care, are an important context for intervention and prevention. For example, research has demonstrated the utility of specialized programs for victims of violence and trauma within medical settings. Campbell and colleagues (2005) review studies examining the effectiveness of Sexual Assault Nurse Examiners (SANE), trained nurses who specialize in providing medical care and evidence collection for sexual assault survivors in hospitals. SANE practitioners pay particular attention to supporting survivors emotionally in the immediate aftermath of the assault. Campbell *et al.*'s review notes the overall effectiveness of these programs, though they highlight the need for more comprehensive evaluation studies.

Other studies have focused on addressing medical settings as a location for identifying trauma survivors and connecting them with a variety of community resources. This work has been mostly focused in three areas: (1) training medical professionals to screen for trauma routinely (particularly for physical intimate partner violence); (2) it also focuses on identifying both the effectiveness of such screening programs, and the challenges and barriers to their widespread implementation; and (3) attitudes of medical personnel to dealing with issues such as interpersonal violence (e.g., Garimella *et al.*, 2000; Minsky-Kelly *et al.*, 2005; Nicolaidis *et al.*, 2005; Stayton and Duncan, 2005; Thurston and Eisener, 2006; Witting *et al.*, 2006). One study by

Borowsky *et al.* (2004) employed a youth violence screening protocol in a pediatric primary care setting and found it to be effective in preventing and reducing the trauma of youth violence. This work highlights primary care as a setting for more primary and secondary prevention of violence in addition to tertiary interventions for survivors.

Finally, trauma can be an impediment to an individual's ability or willingness to obtain routine important medical care and health maintenance check-ups. For example, although trauma survivors report more use of medical services (e.g., Kendall-Tackett, 2003; Ullman and Brecklin, 2003), the literature also contains examples of ways in which medical procedures themselves can trigger memories of traumatic events that have affected one's body (e.g., Coons *et al.*, 2004), experiences that may act as barriers to trauma survivors seeking care. In addition, a study by Plichta *et al.* (1996) found greater dissatisfaction with physicians among women who were survivors of intimate partner violence.

THE IMPACT OF HEALTH CARE PROVIDERS' ATTITUDES

Attitudes of medical professionals to trauma survivors may play a key role here. Campbell and colleagues (1999) examined the impact of responses by medical, legal, and mental health system professionals on rape survivors' mental health. Their study sought to assess the role of broader community resources on the consequences of sexual assault. Of particular importance, their study found that posttraumatic stress disorder was highest among rape survivors who encountered what Campbell *et al.* termed "secondary victimization" (1999, p. 847) from community service providers (including victim blaming attitudes, being subjected to protocols or procedures without explanation, or being told their case wasn't serious enough).

Professionals in medical settings are a key component of the broader community response to trauma survivors, responses that can promote recovery or enhance negative outcomes. Given this, a growing number of studies have begun examining attitudes of

medical professionals about working with certain types of
trauma survivors, particularly survivors of intimate partner
violence, documenting perceived challenges and the need for
specialized training to increase empathy for survivors and skill in
assisting them (e.g., Garimella *et al.*, 2000; Nicolaidis *et al.*,
2005).

GENDER AS A MODERATOR: SETTING A FUTURE RESEARCH AGENDA

While the summary of research above highlights the many
reasons for attending to trauma in the context of primary care,
the majority of studies on which the summary is based have
focused on samples of women and issues of women's health.
The sections that follow examine the important reasons for this
focus, but also explore the utility of using a similar analysis to
describe the health of male trauma survivors.

DEFINING THE LENS OF GENDER

It may be helpful to begin with definitions of terms. Gender is a
term that is often used interchangeably with the term "sex," and
is associated with biological or physiological differences between
males and females. Scholars in the field of gender studies,
however, argue for the separation of these terms (e.g., Gentile,
1998; Unger and Crawford, 1998). They related gender to the
broader context of society and cultural expectations about roles,
behaviors, and attitudes that are separately ascribed as
appropriate for men or women. Gender then becomes more
than simply a physiological marker; rather, it signifies a set of
socialization experiences, a social identity with varying degrees of
access or lack of access to resources or power. It also specifies
potential societal prescriptions about what behaviors or roles are
appropriate for a given individual. A number of theorists
encourage these more complex considerations. For example,
Hare-Mustin and Marecek (1990) highlight the dangers of two
traps into which we can fall: an exclusive focus on gender
similarity or gender difference. In relation to trauma research

more specifically, Humphreys *et al.* (2005) remind us to attend to the complexity of factors related to moderator variables in understanding the consequences of violence. They discuss specifically the role of race, ethnicity, and culture which may interact with:

> **systemic discrimination and bias in the health care, criminal justice, and to a lesser extent, the advocacy systems that have contributed to the differences in responses that we sometimes mistakenly attribute to ethnic or cultural characteristics of victims and perpetrators.**
>
> **(Humphreys *et al.*, 2005, p. 184)**

Gender also seems to be an important and potentially complicating factor when trying to understand trauma and its consequences, and mediating mechanisms.

WHY GENDER MAY BE A SIGNIFICANT MODERATOR:
THE CASE OF GENDER DIFFERENCE

As I described earlier, the field has importantly focused on links between trauma and women's health. This may be the case for a number of reasons. First, to date, one of the larger areas of research on trauma and health examines the relationship between the specific trauma of sexual abuse and outcomes (e.g., Ullman and Brecklin, 2003). Women are disproportionately survivors of sexual assault both in childhood and adulthood. Thus it makes sense to use women's lives as the objects of study for such links. The example of child sexual abuse is illustrative. Research shows that females are disproportionately victims of this form of family violence, with estimates that one in four women have experienced CSA (Edwards *et al.*, 2005), compared to 4 percent to 16 percent of men (e.g., Holmes and Slap (1998) for a review). Flett *et al.*'s (2002) community sample found that more women reported exposure to crime-related trauma than men.

Another important area of research has been the impact of screening for intimate partner violence in medical settings (e.g., Stayton and Duncan, 2005 for a review). Again, given women's disproportionate experience of the more severe forms of this type of trauma, including the experience of physical injury, a focus on this form of intervention in women's lives makes sense. In addition, many of the illnesses that first became the object of study of trauma in their etiology (e.g., irritable bowel syndrome, fibromyalgia, and chronic pain syndromes) are more prevalent among women (see Kendall-Tackett, 2003 for a review). Women also have unique health concerns related specifically to gynecological health that have been shown to be linked to trauma exposure, including the role of sexual assault in risk for STDs and unintended pregnancy, and the greater prevalence of childhood abuse, violent crime victimization, and intimate partner violence among women reporting gynecological problems (e.g., Campbell and Soeken, 1999; Plichta and Abraham, 1996).

Growing numbers of studies, however, also document links between trauma exposure and negative physical health consequences for men (e.g., Flett *et al.*, 2002; Pimlott-Kubiak and Cortina, 2003). Yet, as mentioned earlier, recent books on the role of psychologists in primary care settings refer to the role of trauma almost exclusively in relation to women's health (e.g., James and Folen, 2005; Poleshuck, 2005). Thus, the remainder of this section will explore questions about the utility of examining gender and potential gender differences in increasing our understanding of trauma and physical health.

MEDIATING PROCESSES
Most recently, research and theory focused on identifying pathways through which trauma exerts its negative effects on physical health (e.g., Kendall-Tackett, 2003 for a review), what Merrill and colleagues (2001) refer to as "third generation studies" (p. 993). This literature, both theoretical and empirical, aims to identify risk factors that explain connections between trauma exposure and physical illness. For example, a growing number of studies document the physiological changes to the

body that can follow trauma exposure and increase vulnerability for a variety of forms of psychological and physical distress – or the body may protect against it (see Kendall-Tackett, 2003 for a review). Indeed, it is the identification of these variables that holds promise for identifying points of intervention and prevention for survivors (e.g., Roche *et al.*, 1999). Yet, to date, there have been few direct investigations of the complex relationships between trauma, mediating processes, gender, and outcomes. The following sections review some of the research on mediators that seem key in links between trauma and outcomes (an extensive list of all mediating processes is beyond the scope of this chapter). Interestingly, they are also variables that theoretical and empirical studies suggest may be experienced differently for men and for women.

COPING PROCESSES

Coping processes are a key mediator in connecting stress exposure to outcomes. Lawler and colleagues (2005) found that greater use of avoidance coping related to the traumatic event (e.g., tried to forget about it) was related to more negative outcomes in their mixed-gender sample of college students. Avoidance coping in relation to health concerns and in relation to traumatic events mediated the relationship between PTSD and physical health outcomes as assessed by functional health and self-reported medical diagnoses.

But coping is also an area in which consideration of gender has been found to be important. For example, Nolen-Hoeksema *et al.* (1987) and Turner and Turner (1999) explain gender differences in risk for depression. They note differences in mediating coping mechanisms, such as rumination or emotional reliance; that is, women are more likely to use rumination or emotional reliance, which may put them at risk for depression. Other research suggests that men and women may differ in the range of coping strategies they have access to depending on their location within contexts of social power, the hypothesis being that broader societal systems of gender inequality and patterns of gender role socialization may make different coping resources more or less available to an individual based on gender and other socio-demographics (e.g., Banyard and Graham-Bermann, 1993). Further investigations of patterns of coping following trauma are needed.

HIGH-RISK BEHAVIORS

Also germane to physical health outcomes, trauma is associated with higher levels of risky health behaviors including smoking, substance use, excess body weight, use of seatbelts, and risky sexual behaviors (e.g., Rodgers *et al.*, 2004). We also know from studies beyond the trauma field that there are gender differences in risky health behaviors like substance use (e.g., Cook, 1998) that may lead to different patterns of physical health outcomes for men and women. Other researchers have highlighted the association of interpersonal violence with hostility, which in turn has well-documented links to such health problems as cardiovascular disease (e.g., Kendall-Tackett, 2003 for a review). Jack (2001) reviews research on women and anger, and discusses gender differences in the experience and expression of this emotion, and concludes that such differences may have health consequences that future research should explore.

DEPRESSION AND PTSD

Finally, an extensive body of research examines the role of mental health outcomes, particularly depression and PTSD, as significant mediating factors between trauma exposure and physical health outcomes (e.g., Ford *et al.*, 2004). Women, in general, have higher rates of PTSD than men following trauma exposure (e.g., Breslau *et al.*, 1999; see Kendall-Tackett, 2003 for a review). Banyard and colleagues (2004) found higher symptom scores for female as compared to male survivors of child sexual abuse on mental health outcomes of anxiety, depression, and defensive avoidance. Several theoretical explanations have been discussed that might explain such differences including gender difference in disclosure of symptoms of distress on self-report measures or differences in how distress is expressed. The broader research literature is inconsistent about to what extent men and women differ in their likelihood or willingness to disclose about symptoms of psychological or physical distress. Dindia and Allen (1992) show some support for the hypothesis that women are more likely to self-disclose mental health symptoms because gender role socialization supports this for women more than for men. Yet other researchers have focused on gender differences in expressions of distress, suggesting that both men and women are affected equally by trauma, but manifest their symptoms in different patterns of distress and thus may be at risk for different disorders as trauma outcomes (e.g., Banyard et al., 2004; Turner and Lloyd, 1995). Further work is needed to more fully examine both the relationships between trauma and psychological distress for men and women and reasons for any differences found.

PROTECTIVE FACTORS
Beyond mediating factors that explain risk for negative outcomes, the trauma field is currently trying to develop a better understanding of protective factors, those processes that enable some trauma survivors to do well or thrive over time (e.g., Banyard and Williams, 2007). Questions can be raised about the extent to which gender impacts the availability or use of various positive resources following trauma. Harvey (1996) presents a complex ecological model of trauma recovery, asserting that each trauma survivor will find their own unique pathway to healing, which may or may not involve assistance from professionals, connections to family or to community, and other intra- and inter-personal resources. Understanding patterns in this complexity will enhance our ability to design interventions that help to build on strengths and help survivors move their lives forward.

To date, however, we know little about the extent to which gender creates one such pattern. For example, numerous studies document the important buffering effect of social support following stress (e.g., Kendall-Tackett, 2003 and Ullman, 1999 for reviews). It has positive effects on mental as well as physical health. More specific to the current discussion, Jonzon and Lindblad (2005) found that among survivors who disclosed about their experiences of child sexual abuse, those who received positive reactions from their current partner had fewer psychosomatic symptoms. In contrast, those who received negative reactions to their disclosure from friends had more. Some research suggests that women are more likely to use social support when dealing with stress and report relationships that include greater intimacy (e.g., Rook, 2001 for a review). This literature would suggest that social support may be a protective factor more readily used by women than by men following trauma.

Social support also has costs. Helgeson and colleagues (Fritz and Helgeson, 1998; Helgeson and Fritz, 2000) describe the difference between being involved in caring for others in a positive relationship that produces health benefits with what they term "unmitigated communion" where one focuses on caring for others to the exclusion of self-care. This latter characteristic, also found at greater levels in women, is associated with negative physical and mental health outcomes.

More research on how these processes impact recovery from trauma using a gender perspective is needed. In a recent study of the impact of the trauma of teen dating violence victimization, for example, some forms of social support, such as from family, were protective for females and not for males, while neighborhood connections and support seemed protective for male survivors (Banyard and Cross, 2008). A study by Benda (2006) of male and female veterans who were homeless and substance abusing found that social support was a stronger protective factor against rehospitalization for women than for men, while job satisfaction was a key factor for men. While the samples for each of these studies are unique, they point to ways in which risk and protective factors may differ by gender as well as to key areas for future research.

GENDER AND DELIVERY OF SERVICES

Finally, there is some exploratory evidence related to gender differences in trauma and health care services. Preliminary data from a clinical sample of military families found that medical professionals were much more likely to ask women than men about violence in the home (Banyard et al., 2005). This is perhaps not surprising, since women are much more likely to experience this type of victimization. However, given the range of other traumas potentially affecting the lives of patients seen in medical practices, more general screening may be useful (e.g., Edwards et al., 2004). Nicolaidis et al. (2005), in their study of a program to increase awareness of and empathy for survivors of intimate partner violence, found that lowest levels of empathy for patients' choices to remain in an abusive relationship were for scenarios involving male victims.

ATTENDING TO GENDER SIMILARITY

Hare-Mustin and Marecek (1990) also caution us, however, against being too quick to assume patterns of gender difference. They argue that while ignoring gender as a factor can be problematic, so too can an overly intense focus on gender difference to the exclusion of other factors. Indeed, there are many instances when groups of men and women from similar socioeconomic status or ethnic groups may have more in common with one another than women differing across these other social identity variables. Thus, analyses of gender should also consider the intersection of gender with other social identity groups and room should be made for exploration of conditions of gender similarity. Their work reminds us of the need for balance in our inquiry and practice.

A variety of research studies show links between trauma exposure and physical health effects for men (e.g., Ford, 2004). For example, Beckham et al. (2003) studied male Vietnam combat veterans. Greater combat exposure was related to higher levels of health problems. Higher levels of PTSD in this sample of men were related to more negative health outcomes. The

Adverse Childhood Experiences Study (Edwards *et al.*, 2005) documented the impact of multiple forms of family violence and trauma on adult physical health outcomes in a large sample of men and women. Across their full sample, greater exposure to adverse events in childhood was linked to both increased risky health behaviors (e.g., smoking, use of substances, risky sexual behaviors) and increased likelihood of having one of the diseases high on the list of causes of mortality in the United States (e.g., heart disease, cancer, diabetes). Their study also indicated that trauma was linked to variety of medical illnesses which are of concern to both men and women (e.g., heart disease, cancer, diabetes). Additional analyses from this study showed that overall, the relationship between childhood trauma and adult physical health was not statistically different for women and men in the sample.

Similarly, Ullman and Siegel (1996) found strong links between trauma and physical health outcomes in a sample of men and women when gender was controlled. Flett *et al.* (2002) found overall that gender was not a significant moderator of the trauma physical health outcome relationship across several measures of symptoms, ratings of health, and indices of physical limitations. Importantly, Ullman and Siegel, and Flett *et al.*, found significant moderating effects for ethnicity, supporting the need to attend not simply to categories such as gender but also to other key aspects of social identity that may impact access to resources including race, class, and so on.

This parallels work on gender, trauma, and mental health that finds many patterns of similarity in the links between trauma and mental health outcomes for female and male survivors (e.g., Banyard *et al.*, 2004; Turner and Lloyd, 1995). Indeed, some researchers suggest that gender similarity may be more the norm in responses to trauma, and that previously documented gender differences may be an artifact of the different forms of trauma to which men and women are typically exposed. For example, Turner and Lloyd's (1995) study of cumulative life stress found different rates of exposure to trauma types (e.g., men are more likely to be exposed to combat trauma, while women are more likely to experience sexual violence with no significant differences on such things as childhood physical abuse). Indeed, they argue for the need to examine the total accumulation of trauma across the life course rather than discrete categories or types.

Research by Pimlott-Kubiak and Cortina (2003) investigated the issue of gender more specifically. They critiqued what they discussed as the "feminine vulnerability" (p. 528) view of data on the impact of trauma, a view which asserts that women are at greater risk for negative outcomes following trauma exposure than men. They cite limits of a variety of previous studies showing higher rates of such things as PTSD among female survivors (e.g., Breslau *et al.*, 1999; Flett *et al.*, 2002). Their critique fits well within what Hare-Mustin and Mareck identify as the tendency to assume or reify gender differences where few exist. Pimlott-Kubiak and Cortina (2003) hypothesized that gender differences in outcomes were actually driven by differences in patterns of types of trauma exposure rather than by true gender differences in outcomes. That is, gender similarities were being masked by third variable differences between men and women, specifically the types of trauma they were exposed to. When they compared men and women within similar clusters of lifetime trauma exposure, they in fact found very few gender differences on outcomes including an index of physical health. Related to this, Banyard and colleagues (2004) studied mental health outcomes in a sample of male and female child sexual abuse survivors. They found similarities between male and female survivors on problematic use of alcohol, suicidal tendencies, and a range of patterns of mental health symptoms.

The take-home message is that trauma is linked to physical health outcomes for both men and women. Thus, there is a need to find ways to integrate an understanding of trauma into primary care using a broader approach that appreciates trauma across the lifespan in all patients' lives.

NEXT STEPS

Clinical psychology has shown a growing interest in primary care consultation. For example, in the past three years, three books have been published by the American Psychological Association on this topic (Frank *et al.*, 2004; Gatchel and Oordt, 2003; James and Folen, 2005). These works review the important roles psychologists are filling within settings historically defined as the locus of treatment for physical health concerns. In this context, trauma has been given attention. For example, all three recent American Psychological Association texts on primary care practice make some reference to trauma. However, its treatment is almost exclusively in relation to female survivors and women's health. For example, in one book it is discussed only in terms of women's health, in another it is not discussed at all, and in the third, while abuse such as sexual assault is listed among the common primary care conditions, the main discussion of violence is in relation to women's health care. The preceding review, highlighting patterns of both gender similarity and difference, suggests the need to also develop screening tools for trauma related to men's health. Indeed, psychologists can help integrate trauma treatment for men into primary care. The earlier review that highlights both the need to attend to areas of similarity and difference is relevant here to recommendations for practice.

The preceding review highlights that to date we understand more about links between physical health and trauma for women. We can learn from this research about the importance of also screening for men's trauma histories in health care settings and conceptualizing integrated trauma and physical health interventions for them. For example, we know from studies of women that trauma can act as a significant barrier to receiving health care as survivors avoid regular medical examinations because they may trigger memories of traumatic events. We know less about the barriers to seeking care for men and this may be an important area for further inquiry. Gender differences and similarities in mediators including risky health behaviors and health-related coping strategies will also suggest areas for future prevention and intervention efforts. For instance, if social support is protective for all but used more often by women, strategies to facilitate social support for male survivors may be helpful. It is not a matter of either/or. Rather, we should emphasize different areas of positive coping or adaptation in developing holistic interventions that treat physical illness in the broader context of psychological distress and coping with trauma.

A continued focus on gender differences also seems in order. In the broader context, women worldwide are more likely to encounter problems accessing health care as recent studies show gender disparity in terms of referral for medical tests and lower health insurance enrollment rates (e.g., Landrine and Klonoff, 2001 for a review). Clearly, women also are uniquely vulnerable to medical problems related to pregnancy, childbirth, and certain types of cancers and sexually transmitted diseases. Thus, the intersection of trauma with these issues will, of necessity, continue to focus on women's health. Women are also differentially exposed to various types of trauma. Women, for example, are more likely to experience sexual assault and, thus, special programs like Sexual Assault Nurse Examiner (SANE) programs that have been shown to be effective (e.g., Campbell *et al.*, 2005) and that may disproportionately serve women are needed. Women are also at disproportionate risk for severe physical intimate partner violence and resultant injuries. Thus, continued training of medical personnel to screen for this problem and research on the effectiveness of such programs is a useful role for psychologists in primary care settings.

Overall we are in a position to treat gender in a unique way in our examination of the intersection of trauma and physical health – not blindly assuming gender similarity, which often results in women being left out of medical research altogether. But also not reifying gender differences, providing ideas for ways in which prevention and intervention techniques may improve overall health care delivery for all survivors.

REFERENCES

Arias, I. (2004). The legacy of child maltreatment: Long-term health consequences for women. *Journal of Women's Health, 13*, 468–473.

Banyard, V.L. and Cross, C. (2008). Consequences of teen dating violence: Understanding intervening variables in ecological context. *Violence Against Women, 14*, 998–1013.

Banyard, V.L. and Graham-Bermann, S.A. (1993). Can women cope? A gender analysis of theories of coping with stress. *Psychology of Women Quarterly, 17*, 303–318.

Banyard, V.L. and Williams, L.M. (2007). Women's voices on recovery: A multi-method study of the complexity of recovery from child sexual abuse. *Child Abuse and Neglect, 31*, 275–290.

Banyard, V.L., Williams, L.M., and Saunders, B. (2005). *Understanding links between trauma and physical health outcomes: Implications for collaboration with primary care settings.* Paper presented at the 9th International Family Violence Research Conference, Portsmouth, New Hampshire, July.

Banyard, V.L., Williams, L.M., and Siegel, J.A. (2004). Childhood sexual abuse: A gender perspective on context and consequences. *Child Maltreatment, 9*, 223–238.

Beckham, J.C., Taft, C.T., Vrana, S.R., Feldman, M.E., Barefoot, J.C., Moore, S.D., Mozley, S.L., Butterfield, M.I., and Calhoun, P.S. (2003). Ambulatory monitoring and physical health report in Vietnam veterans with and without chronic Posttraumatic Stress Disorder. *Journal of Traumatic Stress, 16*, 329–335.

Benda, B.B. (2006). Survival analysis of social support and trauma among homeless male and female veterans who abuse substances. *American Journal of Orthopsychiatry, 76*, 70–79.

Borowsky, I.W., Mozayeny, S., Stuenkel, K., and Ireland, M. (2004). Effects of a primary care-based intervention on violence behavior and injury in children. *Pediatrics, 114*, 392–399.

Breslau, N., Chilcoat, H.D., Kessler, R.C., and Davis, G.C. (1999). Previous exposure to trauma and PTSD effects of subsequent trauma: Results from the Detroit area survey of trauma. *American Journal of Psychiatry, 156*, 902–907.

Campbell, J.C., and Soeken, K.L. (1999). Forced sex and intimate partner violence: Effects on women's risk and women's health. *Violence Against Women, 5*, 1017–1035.

Campbell, R., Patterson, D., and Lichty, L.F. (2005). The effectiveness of sexual assault nurse examiner (SANE) programs. *Trauma, Violence, and Abuse, 6*, 313–329.

Campbell, R., Sefl, T., Barnes, H.E., Ahrens, C. E., Wasco, S.M., and Zaragoza-Diesfield, Y. (1999). Community services for rape survivors: Enhancing psychological well-being or increasing trauma? *Journal of Consulting and Clinical Psychology, 67*, 847–858.

Cook. E.P. (1998). Gender and psychological distress. In D.L. Anselmi and A.L. Law (eds), *Questions of Gender: Perspectives and Paradoxes* (pp. 740–747). Boston, MA: McGraw-Hill.

Coons, H.L., Morgenstern, D., Hoffman, E.M., Striepe, M.I., and Buch, C. (2004). Psychologists in women's primary care and obstetrics-gynecology: Consultation and treatment issues. In R.G. Frank, S.H. McDaniel, J.H. Bray, and M. Heldring (eds), *Primary Care Psychology* (pp. 209–226). Washington, DC: American Psychological Association.

Dindia, K. and Allen, M. (1992). Sex differences in self-disclosure: A meta-analysis. *Psychological Bulletin, 112*, 106–124.

Edwards, V.J., Anda, R.F., Felitti, V.J., and Dube, S.R. (2004). Adverse childhood experiences and health-related quality of life as an adult. In K. Kendall-Tackett (ed.), *Health Consequences of Abuse in the Family* (pp. 81–94). Washington, DC: American Psychological Association.

Edwards, V.J., Anda, R.F., Dube, S.R., Dong, M., Chapman, D.P., and Felitti, V.J. (2005). The wide-ranging health outcomes of adverse childhood experiences. In K. Kendall-Tackett and S. Giacomoni (eds), *Child Victimization* (pp. 8–16). Kingston, NJ: Civic Research Institute.

Felitti, V.J., Anda, R.F., Nordenberg, D., Williamson, D.F., Spitz, A.M., Edwards, V.J., Koss, M.P., and Marks, J.S. (1998). Relationship of childhood abuse and household dysfunction to many of the leading causes of death in adults. *American Journal of Preventive Medicine, 14*, 245–258.

Flett, R.A., Kazantzis, N., Long, N.R., MacDonald, C., and Millar, M. (2002). Traumatic events and physical health in a New Zealand community sample. *Journal of Traumatic Stress, 15*, 303–312.

Ford, D.E. (2004) Depression, trauma, and cardiovascular health. Preview. In P.P. Schnurr and B.L. Green (eds), *Trauma and Health: Physical Health Consequences of Exposure to Extreme Stress* (pp. 73–97). Washington, DC: American Psychological Association.

Ford, J.D., Schnurr, P.P., Friedman, M.J., Green, B.L., Adams, G., and Jex, S. (2004). Posttraumatic stress disorder symptoms, physical health, and health care utilization 50 years after repeated exposure to a toxic gas. *Journal of Traumatic Stress, 17*, 185–194.

Frank, R.G., McDaniel, S.H., Bray, J.H., and Heldring, M. (eds) (2004). *Primary Care Psychology*. Washington, DC: American Psychological Association.

Fritz, H.L., and Helgeson, V.S. (1998). Distinctions of unmitigated communion from communion: Self-neglect and overinvolvement with others. *Journal of Personality and Social Psychology, 75*, 121–140.

Garimella, R., Plichta, S.B., Hourseman, C., and Garzon, L. (2000). Physician beliefs about victims of spouse abuse and about the physician role. *Journal of Women's Health and Gender-based Medicine, 9*, 405–411.

Gatchel, R.J., and Oordt, M.S. (2003). *Clinical Health Psychology and Primary Care*. Washington, DC: American Psychological Association.

Gentile, D.A. (1998). Just what are sex and gender, anyway? A call for a new terminological standard. In D.L. Anselmi and A.L. Law (eds), *Questions of Gender* (pp.14–17). Boston, MA: McGraw-Hill.

Hare-Mustin, R.T. and Marecek, J. (eds) (1990). *Making a Difference: Psychology and the Construction of Gender*. New Haven, CT: Yale University Press.

Harvey, M. (1996). An ecological view of psychological trauma and trauma recovery. *Journal of Traumatic Stress, 9*, 3–23.

Helgeson, V.S. and Fritz, H.L. (2000). The implications of unmitigated agency and unmitigated communion for domains of problem behavior. *Journal of Personality, 68*, 1031–1057.

Holmes, W.C. and Slap, G.B. (1998). Sexual abuse of boys: Definition, prevalence, correlates, sequelae, and management. *JAMA: Journal of the American Medical Association, 280*, 1855–1862.

Humphreys, J., Sharps, P.W., and Campbell, J.C. (2005). What we know and what we still need to learn. *Journal of Interpersonal Violence, 20*, 182–187.

Jack, D.C. (2001). Anger. In J. Worell (ed.), *Encyclopedia of Women and Gender* (pp.137–147). San Diego, CA: Academic Press.

James, L.C., and Folen, R.A. (2005). *The Primary Care Consultant*. Washington, DC: American Psychological Association.

Jonzon, E., and Lindblad, F. (2005). Adult female victims of child sexual abuse: Multitype maltreatment and disclosure characteristics related to subjective health. *Journal of Interpersonal Violence, 20*, 651–666.

Kendall-Tackett, K. (2003). *Treating the Lifetime Health Effects of Childhood Victimization*. Kingston, NJ: Civic Research Institute.

Kendall-Tackett, K. (ed.) (2004). *Health Consequences of Abuse in the Family*. Washington, DC: American Psychological Association.

Landrine, H. and Klonoff, E.A. (2001). Health and healthcare: How gender makes women sick. In J. Worell (ed.), *Encyclopedia of Women and Gender* (pp. 577–592). San Diego, CA: Academic Press.

Lang, A.J., Rodgers, C.S., Laffaye, C., Satz, L.E., Dresselhaus, T.R., and Stein, M.B. (2003). Sexual trauma, Posttraumatic Stress Disorder, and health behavior. *Behavioral Medicine, 28*, 150–159.

Lawler, C., Ouimette, P., and Dahlstedt, D. (2005). Posttraumatic stress symptoms, coping, and physical health status among university students seeking health care. *Journal of Traumatic Stress, 18*, 741–750.

Merrill, L.L., Thomsen, C.J., Sinclair, B.B., Gold, S.R., and Milner, J.S. (2001). Predicting the impact of child sexual abuse on women: The role of abuse severity, parental support, and coping strategies. *Journal of Consulting and Clinical Psychology, 69*, 992–1006.

Minsky-Kelly, D., Hamberger, L.K., Paper, D.A., and Wolff, M. (2005). We've had training, now what? Qualitative analysis of barriers to domestic violence screening and referral in a health care setting. *Journal of Interpersonal Violence, 20*, 1288–1309.

Nicolaidis, C., Curry, M., and Gerrity, M. (2005). Measuring the impact of the Voices of Survivors program on health care workers' attitudes toward survivors of intimate partner violence. *Journal of General Internal Medicine, 20*, 731–737.

Nicolaidis, C., Curry, M., McFarland, B., and Gerrity, M. (2004). Violence, mental health, and physical symptoms in an academic internal medicine practice. *Journal of General Internal Medicine, 19*, 819–827.

Nolen-Hoeksema, S., Larson, J., and Grayson, C. (1999). Explaining the gender difference in depressive symptoms. *Journal of Personality and Social Psychology, 77*, 1061–1072.

Pimlott-Kubiak, S., and Cortina, L.M. (2003). Gender, victimization, and outcomes: Reconceptualizing risk. *Journal of Consulting and Clinical Psychology, 71*, 528–539.

Plichta, S.B., and Falik, M. (2001). Prevalence of violence and its implications for women's health. *Women's Health Issues, 11*, 244–258.

Plichta, S.B. and Abraham, C. (1996). Violence and gynecologic health in women > 50 years old. *American Journal of Obstetrics And Gynecology, 174*, 903–907.

Plichta, S.B., Duncan, M.M., and Plichta, L. (1996). Spouse abuse, patient-physician communication, and patient satisfaction. *American Journal of Preventive Medicine, 12*, 297–303.

Poleshuck, E.L. (2005). Women's health and the role of primary care psychology. In L.C. James and R.A. Folen, *The Primary Care Consultant* (pp. 217–241). Washington, DC: American Psychological Association.

Roche, D.N., Runtz, M.G., and Hunter, M.A. (1999). Adult attachment: A mediator between child sexual abuse and later psychological adjustment. *Journal of Interpersonal Violence, 14*, 184–207.

Rodgers, C.S., Lang, A.J., Laffaye, C., Satz, L.E., Dresselhaus, T.R., and Stein, M.B. (2004). The impact of individual forms of childhood maltreatment on health behavior. *Child Abuse and Neglect, 28*, 575–586.

Rook, K.S. (2001). Social support. In J. Worell (ed.), *Encyclopedia of Women and Gender* (pp.1079–1089). San Diego, CA: Academic Press.

Stayton, C.D., and Duncan, M.M. (2005). Mutable influences on intimate partner abuse screening in health care settings. *Trauma, Violence, and Abuse, 6*, 271–285.

Thurston, W.E. and Eisener, A.C. (2006). Successful integration and maintenance of screening for domestic violence in the health sector. *Trauma, Violence, and Abuse, 7*, 83–92.

Turner, R.J., and Lloyd, D.A. (1995). Lifetime traumas and mental health: The significance of cumulative adversity. *Journal of Health and Social Behavior, 36*, 360–376.

Turner, H.A. and Turner, R.J. (1999). Gender, social status, and emotional reliance. *Journal of Health and Social Behavior, 40*, 360–373.

Ullman, S. (1999). Social support and recovery from sexual assault: A review. *Aggression and Violent Behavior, 4*, 343–358.

Ullman, S., and Brecklin, L.R. (2003). Sexual assault history and health-related outcomes in a national sample of women. *Psychology of Women Quarterly, 27*, 46–57.

Ullman, S., and Siegel, J.M. (1996). Traumatic events and physical health in a community sample. *Journal of Traumatic Stress, 9*, 703–720.

Unger, R.K. and Crawford, M. (1998). Commentary: Sex and gender – the troubled relationship between terms and concepts. In D.L. Anselmi and A.L. Law (eds), *Questions of Gender* (pp.18–21). Boston, MA: McGraw-Hill.

Witting, M.D., Furuno, J.P., Hirshon, J.M., Kurgman, S.D., and Perisse, A.R.S. (2006). Support for emergency department screening for intimate partner violence depends on perceived risk. *Journal of Interpersonal Violence, 21*, 585–596.

Thinking outside the box

Why research on self-efficacy and sleep disorders is relevant for trauma survivors

Kathleen A. Kendall-Tackett

_____

IN PREVIOUS CHAPTERS, the authors outlined some practical ways that trauma practice may be integrated into primary care. In this chapter I explore two additional areas that are rarely, if ever, integrated into treatment plans for trauma survivors. These are a patient's self-efficacy and the quality of their sleep. I selected these two areas to focus on because of the strong relation each has to health, and trauma negatively affects both. Often, these two issues are not even assessed, let alone addressed. Yet research suggests that addressing them is likely to make a substantial difference in improving the health of trauma survivors. The first area I describe is self-efficacy.

SELF-EFFICACY

Self-efficacy refers to how competent people feel they are. These beliefs influence the course of action a person chooses, how much effort is put into the action, how long she perseveres, and how much she accomplishes (Bandura, 1999). Someone who is high in self-efficacy persists in the face of difficulty and puts forth more effort. In contrast, someone who is low in self-efficacy often quits in the face of difficulty, is more likely to attribute failure to some flaw within themselves, and is likely to be anxious or depressed (McAuley and Courneya, 1993). Self-efficacy is often assessed by asking participants to answer questions about how much confidence they have that they can affect change in their lives.

THE ORIGIN OF SELF-EFFICACY

According to attachment theory, self-efficacy is influenced by the quality of attachment a child has with his primary caregiver. This caregiver provides the "safe base" from which the child gains mastery experience. Children with secure attachments learn that they can get their needs met through their own efforts. In contrast, when children are abused or neglected, and their attachments insecure, they grow up believing that their efforts are ineffective, and they must rely on others who may or may not meet their needs (Weinberg et al., 1999).

In a study of children ages 8 to 12, Toth and Cicchetti (1996) found that physically abused and neglected children believed they were less competent than their non-maltreated peers. These beliefs were present on three different dimensions: scholastic competence, social acceptance, and behavioral conduct. The children's relationships with their mothers served to either buffer or exacerbate these effects.

In a study of college students, both self-efficacy and self-esteem were related to family climate and the parents' childrearing style. An affectionless parental rearing style accounted for 13 percent of the variance in self-efficacy, self-esteem, and depression (Oliver and Paull, 1995).

Sexually risky behavior is also related to self-efficacy. In a sample of 100 teens admitted to a psychiatric hospital, 38 percent had been sexually abused. The sexually abused teens had significantly lower self-efficacy concerning condom use; abuse history accounted for 16 percent of the variance in condom-use self-efficacy. The authors concluded that a history of sexual abuse impairs safe-sex decision-making ability (Brown et al., 1997). These researchers found similar results in another group of teenage girls. In this study, girls who had been sexually abused showed significantly less condom self-efficacy, had less knowledge of HIV, and also had significantly higher rates of HIV infection (Brown *et al.*, 2000). Self-efficacy was also a factor in revictimization. In a longitudinal study of 8th and 9th grade girls, Walsh and Foshee (1998) found that low self-efficacy predicted whether the girls had been forced into sexual activity in the six months between assessments.

Ryan and colleagues found that a dysfunctional family may block college students' future job prospects. The family may not model functional coping in general, and they may be excessively negative and discouraging, which can impact self-efficacy in seeking a job (Ryan *et al.*, 1996). In contrast, family support was related to stronger self-efficacy beliefs in a study of Latino college students' adjustment to college. Students who had higher self-efficacy were more strongly persistent in their intentions. Strength of intentions also had an indirect association with better health (Torres and Solberg, 2001).

The studies sited above indicate that trauma can lead to low self-efficacy. But the relationship between self-efficacy and trauma appears to be bidirectional in that low self-efficacy can increase the risk of developing posttraumatic stress disorder (PTSD) following exposure to a traumatic event. In a prospective study of firefighters, high hostility and low self-efficacy at baseline accounted for 42 percent of the variance in PTSD symptoms two years later. Subjects who had both high hostility and low self-efficacy were at increased risk for depression, anxiety, general psychological morbidity, and global symptom severity (Heinrichs *et al.*, 2005).

Most of the studies specifically examining the impact of trauma on self-efficacy have been from the child maltreatment field. But other trauma-producing events can also undermine a victim's beliefs about their ability to control their lives, as Koss (1990, p. 376) describes.

Victimization activates negative self-images such that victims see themselves as weak, needy, frightened, and

out of control. . . . Visions of the self as healthy, active, or strong may be necessary to regain a convincing sense of control.

SELF-EFFICACY AND HEALTH

Not surprisingly, patients who are high in self-efficacy are often healthier than those with low self-efficacy. Researchers have found that self-efficacy influences adaptation to disability, compliance with treatment, and health behaviors. These studies are briefly summarized below.

ADAPTATION TO DISABILITY AND CHRONIC CONDITIONS

Self-efficacy was related to compliance with medication and exercise regimens for people with rheumatoid arthritis (Marks, 2001). In another study, rheumatoid-arthritis (RA) patients who had low self-efficacy were more fatigued than RA patients who were high in self-efficacy (Jump *et al.*, 2004). Moreover, self-efficacy was related to pain and well-being, and was a potent predictor of health status overall.

For patients recovering from surgery, self-efficacy predicted recovery, even after controlling for prior health, functional limitations, sex and age, optimism, health value (the importance the person placed on their health), and perceived health competence (Waldrop *et al.*, 2001). Self-efficacy was also related to recovery from orthopedic surgery. A study of patients after joint-replacement surgery found that self-efficacy at three months independently predicted disability at nine months, even after controlling for pre-surgery and three-month disability level (Orbell *et al.*, 2001).

Self-efficacy significantly predicted survival in a study of patients with chronic obstructive pulmonary disease (Kaplan *et al.*, 1994), and recovery from coronary bypass surgery. Patients with high self-efficacy were more compliant with post-operative use of the incentive spirometer, had shorter ICU stays, and shorter hospital stays overall (Mahler and Kulik, 1998).

COMPLIANCE WITH TREATMENT

Compliance with treatment is another key factor in health – especially for people with chronic conditions. In a study of physiotherapy for urinary incontinence, women with high self-efficacy were more likely to adhere to the recommended treatment regimen (Alewijnse et al., 2001). Self-efficacy was also related to adherence to a weekly regimen of Interferon beta-1a for relapsing multiple sclerosis (Mohr et al., 2001).

Type-2 diabetes is an illness with a strong behavioral component; those who don't comply with treatment are often subject to life-threatening complications. In a study of patients with diabetes, those with high-perceived control were significantly less likely to be depressed or anxious, had better blood glucose control, and fewer microvascular complications, such as retinopathy, neuropathy, and kidney disease (Macrodimitris and Endler, 2001).

In HIV treatment, medical adherence is also vital to success. In a study of 71 men and women who were on rigorous treatment regimens for HIV, 31 percent had missed at least one dose in the preceding five days. This is significant because even one missed dose can diminish the effectiveness of treatment. Depression, low self-efficacy, and lack of social support were all related to poor treatment compliance (Catz et al., 2000). In another study of patients with HIV/AIDS, self-efficacy at Time 1 increased medication adherence three months later and subsequent viral load six months later. Depression and hopelessness were both identified as factors related to low adherence (Simoni et al., 2006).

HEALTH BEHAVIORS

Self-efficacy is a predictor of health-enhancing behaviors (Wallston, 2001). In a study of 11,632 patients in Wales, participants who believed that they controlled their own health performed a greater number of health-enhancing behaviors, whereas those who believed that their health was due to fate or chance were less likely to participate in health-enhancing behaviors (Norman *et al.*, 1998). In a review of the literature, people high in self-efficacy were more likely to adhere to an exercise program (McAuley and Courneya, 1993), and subjects with high self-efficacy had lower heart rates, systolic and diastolic blood pressure and skin temperature in response to a stressor (Sanz and Villamarin, 2001).

Depression, a problem that tends to co-occur with low self-efficacy, is also related to reduced behaviors that undermined health. In a study of black and white adolescent females (ages 16 to 18), Franko *et al.* (2005) found that teens who were depressed at Time 1 were more likely to be smokers, had more eating concerns, a lower level of education, and lower self-worth than their non-depressed counterparts when assessed three years later.

INTERVENTIONS TO INCREASE SELF-EFFICACY

From the above-cited studies, it is clear that low self-efficacy can lead to poor health. If self-efficacy increases health-enhancing behaviors, then it is desirable to try to increase it in trauma survivors. Fortunately, some interventions have proven effective in increasing self-efficacy. These interventions appear promising for trauma survivors, and are likely to improve their health.

PATIENT EDUCATION

Patient education is an important technique to improve self-efficacy. In their qualitative study of why HIV patients were not complying with treatment, Siegel *et al.* (1999) discovered that there were often logical reasons, from these patients' perspectives, for their non-compliance. For example, many of these patients were modifying their treatment regimens when they perceived that the medications were not alleviating their symptoms, or were even increasing their symptoms. More alarming, the patients were not informing their doctors about these alterations, which included reductions of dose, or "drug holidays." The authors encouraged physicians to educate patients about the dangers of these unauthorized modifications to their treatment regimens and to teach patients some strategies to cope with medication side-effects. But they also encouraged physicians to understand that patients who made these modifications did care about their health. In essence, they were trying to gain some mastery over their own health, albeit in an ineffective way.

Patient education was also found to be important in a study of patients with fibromyalgia (Dobkin *et al.*, 2005). In this study, patients were assigned to an exercise program. The authors found that high treatment adherence during the study predicted maintenance of the exercise program after the study ended. Since exercise is an important part of treatment for fibromyalgia, the authors recommended patient education in combination with cognitive-behavioral therapy (CBT) to increase adherence to treatment in future studies. They felt that CBT would help patients minimize catastrophizing about bodily sensations when exercising, and would also address their mental barriers to exercising.

PROXY EFFICACY

Related to patient education is a construct known as proxy efficacy (Bray and Cowan, 2004). This refers to the confidence patients have that professionals can function effectively on their behalf. With proxy efficacy, patients believe that their care providers are competent and capable of providing care. Patients' proxy-efficacy beliefs increase their self-efficacy for programs such as exercise after cardiac rehabilitation.

Bray and Cowan (2004) exhort health care providers to inspire confidence in their patients. If care providers tell their patients that they are confident the patients can carry out the exercises needed to get better, the patients are more likely to do so. And if they do so, they can improve their health.

COMPLIANCE WITH TREATMENT

One of the best ways to increase self-efficacy is through performance accomplishments – actually doing the behavior that is part of the treatment regimen. In a study of patients with Type-2 diabetes, adherence to treatment influenced self-efficacy. The patients who were less adherent had lower self-efficacy, a higher body mass index, and were more depressed (Sacco et al., 2005). Improved self-efficacy increased low-income mothers' consumption of fruits and vegetables (Langenberg et al., 2000), and after participating in an exercise program, older adults had improved self-efficacy and improved body parameters. These contributed to increased self-worth six months later (McAuley et al., 2000).

WRITING ABOUT STRESSFUL EXPERIENCES
Another promising intervention that helps people gain mastery over their experiences is writing about them. Gaining mastery over experiences is another way to increase self-efficacy (Jones et al., 2004). In a study of patients with asthma or rheumatoid-arthritis (Smyth et al., 1999), patients who wrote about emotionally stressful situations had measurably improved symptoms at four months. Symptom severity was rated by a physician. The group assigned to write about neutral topics did not improve.

Another study used writing to alter women with HIV's level of optimism (Mann, 2001). Women who were pessimistic at the beginning of the study were assigned to write about a positive future for themselves, or they were assigned to a no-writing condition. As predicted, women in the writing condition increased their optimism, adherence to treatment, and their tolerance of medication side-effects.

CONCLUSIONS
Traumatic events can shatter people's beliefs about who they are and how competent they are. If people believe that they are powerless to effect any positive change in their lives, they are less likely to behave in health-enhancing ways. However, if patients increase their self-efficacy, they are more likely to behave in healthy ways, and will cope more effectively with any chronic condition they may have.

In the following section, I describe the impact of traumatic events on sleep. Sleep is vital to health, but is often seriously undermined in the wake of trauma. By improving sleep quality, we can dramatically enhance the health of trauma survivors.

SLEEP DIFFICULTIES

Trauma survivors often have poor quality of sleep. This is another way that trauma can impact health. Yet, as a field, we have underestimated the impact of traumatic events on sleep. In this section, I describe what we know so far about sleep difficulties for trauma survivors, why these difficulties are relevant to health, and what some effective treatment approaches are.

WHAT IS A SLEEP DISORDER?

Sleep disorders cover a wide range of problems. Some of these disorders can be measured via patient questionnaire. Other sleep difficulties need to be measured via polysomnographic studies. Polysomnographic studies are necessary to detect common problems, such as sleep-disordered breathing (e.g., sleep apneas), and sleep-movement disorders (e.g., restless leg syndrome). Sleep disorders can be grouped into three broad categories. These are listed below.

- *Insomnia*. Insomnia is the best known of the sleep disorders, and often the only one researchers even ask about. It refers to someone's inability to either fall asleep or stay asleep, and it is often precipitated by life stress, worry, and depression. Insomnia may also be caused by lifestyle factors (e.g., daytime napping, excessive caffeine consumption).
- *Hypersomnia*. This refers to excessive daytime sleepiness and is a symptom associated with conditions such as sleep apnea.
- *Parasomnias*. Parasomnias are unusual behaviors that occur during sleep. These include sleep-walking, bruxism (teeth grinding), and most relevant to our discussion, nightmares, which occur during REM sleep.

HOW TRAUMA INFLUENCES SLEEP

Trauma has a substantial impact on sleep. In one community sample, 68 percent sexual abuse survivors reported having sleep difficulties, with 45 percent having repetitive nightmares (Teegan, 1999). Thirty-three percent of teens who had been raped indicated that they "slept badly" compared with 16 percent of the non-assaulted comparison group. Of the assaulted teens, 28 percent had nightmares (compared with 11 percent), and 56 percent woke during the night (compared with 21 percent; Choquet et al., 1997).

Hulme (2000) found that sleep problems among sexual abuse survivors were common in a primary care sample. Fifty-two percent of sexual abuse survivors reported that they could not sleep at night (compared with 24 percent of the non-abused group), and 36 percent reported nightmares (compared with 13 percent). Intrusive symptoms were also common with 53 percent of sexual abuse survivors reporting sudden thoughts or images of past events (compared with 18 percent of the non-abused group).

In another study, subjects who had experienced physical abuse, emotional abuse, sexual abuse, neglect, medical trauma, or a combination of these events reported significantly more sleep difficulties than the group with no trauma. These difficulties included nightmares, sleep apnea, and narcolepsy (Chambers and Belicki, 1998). In another study, difficulty sleeping and feeling tired were twice as likely in abuse survivors recruited from a gastroenterology practice than their non-abused counterparts (Leserman et al., 1998).

In a sample of battered women living in shelters (N = 50), 70 percent reported poor sleep quality, 28 percent went to bed very fatigued, and 40 percent woke up feeling very fatigued (Humphreys et al., 1999). Moreover, 82 percent described one or more of the following characteristics of disturbed sleep: many wakings over the course of the night, restless sleep, and early-morning waking. Six described vivid nightmares that included recent incidents of abuse. Women with children reported more sleep problems than women without children, as the women with children were more likely to worry about them.

In a study of sleep disorders in sexual assault survivors, 80 percent had either sleep-breathing or sleep-movement disorders. Both of these disorders were linked to higher levels of depression and suicidality, and women who had both types of sleep disorders had the most severe symptoms. The authors speculated that fragmented sleep potentiated the symptoms for women after a sexual assault, stretching their fragile coping abilities to breaking point (Krakow et al., 2000).

SLEEP AND PSYCHOPATHOLOGY

At this time, the relationship between sleep disorders and psychopathology is unclear. We know that they co-occur because sleep problems are common among people with psychiatric disorders, affecting anywhere from 50 percent to 80 percent of psychiatric patients (compared to 7.5 percent of people without a psychiatric disorder; Morin and Ware, 1996).

Some trauma practitioners assume that sleep problems are merely a symptom of an underlying psychiatric condition. They also assume that once they have dealt with the underlying depression, anxiety or PTSD, sleep will also improve. This is not necessarily a safe assumption. What more recent thinking on this topic indicates is that sleep problems are often comorbid disorders rather than merely symptoms. If practitioners address the sleep problems, the co-occurring psychiatric disorders often improve, even when not directly treated (Krakow et al., 2000; Roberts et al., 2000). In this section, I explore the relationship between sleep disturbance and three common psychiatric sequelae of traumatic events.

ANXIETY

Fuller and colleagues (1997) found that anxiety was related to several key alterations in sleep. High-anxiety subjects took longer to fall asleep, had a smaller percentage of slow-wave sleep, had more frequent transitions into light sleep, and a greater percentage of light sleep. These patients also had more early micro-arousals, and lower REM density compared to subjects who were low in anxiety.

In another study, anxiety over current relationships was related to sleep difficulties. In this study, men and women who were anxious about their attachments to their spouses had more self-reported sleep difficulties (Carmichael and Reis, 2005). This finding was true even after controlling for depression. The author speculated that a pattern of insecure attachments may have started during childhood and was now spilling over into adult relationships. These relational problems were manifesting themselves as sleep difficulties.

DEPRESSION

Sleep difficulties are also related to depression. Data from a large sample of older adults (N = 2,370) indicated that sleep disorders were strongly associated with the risk of major depression. Early-morning waking was the sleep disturbance most consistently related to depression over time (Roberts et al., 2000).

Sleep difficulties also predicted a longer course of depression. In a ten-year study of outcomes of depression treatment, those with severe fatigue and trouble sleeping were more likely to have a chronic course of depression (Moos and Cronkite, 1999). Nicassio and Wallston (1992) investigated the link between sleep, pain, and depression in patients with rheumatoid-arthritis. Data were collected twice during a two-year period. High rates of pain and sleep problems were associated with depression at both Times 1 and 2. The authors concluded that pain may make sleep problems worse in RA patients, and both pain and sleep difficulties may contribute to depression over time.

Depression also impacts sleep architecture. Sleep architecture refers to the percentage of time people spend in various sleep stages and the distribution of those stages throughout the night (Morin and Ware, 1996). The alteration most likely in depressed individuals is an alteration of REM sleep parameters. Specifically, depressed people are more likely to have longer periods of REM earlier in the night than non-depressed people (referred to as a "short REM latency"). They are also likely to have increased percentages of REM sleep and less deep sleep as a result (Morin and Ware, 1996).

One study examined the strength of the relationship between sleep architecture and depression (Perlis *et al.*, 1997). Using canonical correlation, the authors found that severe depression drastically reduces the amount of time spent in Stage 4 (delta) sleep. Further, depressed patients have more REM sleep, and REM sleep occurs earlier in the night (Perlis *et al.*, 1997; Ware and Morin, 1997). Antidepressants, particularly tricyclics and MAO inhibitors, decrease percentage of REM sleep and prolong the latency to first REM sleep. Cognitive-behavioral therapy may also produce these changes (Ware and Morin, 1997).

POSTTRAUMATIC STRESS DISORDER (PTSD)

Sleep disorders are also common in PTSD, with disturbed sleep and nightmares being key symptoms (Morin and Ware, 1996). PTSD also appears to have a relationship to REM latency, but this relationship is unclear. Some survivors have a shortened REM latency, while others have a lengthened REM latency. The reaction of a particular trauma survivor tends to vary by both the recency of the traumatic event and the severity of current PTSD (Morin and Ware, 1996).

Sleep problems may also keep symptoms of PTSD active. In a study of 23 patients who suffered from chronic nightmares and obstructive sleep apnea, patients who had completed a treatment program for their sleep problems (N = 14) were compared with patients who had dropped out of the program (N = 9). Twenty-one months later, those who completed the program had substantially improved sleep compared with those who had not. Of the patients with nightmares, a subset also had a diagnosis of PTSD. When the patients with PTSD were compared with the PTSD/no-treatment patients, those in the treatment group had 75 percent improvement in their PTSD symptoms. In contrast, the six patients in the PTSD/no-treatment group reported a 43 percent worsening of symptoms. The authors concluded that treating the sleep difficulties appeared to also improve PTSD symptoms, and went on to recommend a full evaluation of sleep in patients with PTSD (Krakow et al., 2000).

HOW SLEEP IMPACTS HEALTH

Poor sleep quality has a profound effect on health. It compromises immune, metabolic, and neuroendocrine function, chronically activates the HPA axis, and even increases mortality risk (Carmichael and Reis, 2005). In a meta-analysis of 19 studies, Pilcher and Huffcutt (1996) found that sleep deprivation strongly impacts functioning in three broad categories: motor functioning, cognitive functioning, and mood. Sleep-deprived subjects performed at a level comparable to the lowest 10 percent of the non-sleep-deprived subjects. Cognitive performance was much more likely to be affected than motor performance. Sleep deprivation leads to memory impairment, diminished concentration, and even interpersonal problems. But the negative impact of sleep deprivation on mood was the most severe of all. Indeed, sleep-deprived subjects reported moods that were three standard deviations lower than their non-sleep-deprived counterparts. Interestingly, partial sleep deprivation was more damaging on all three types of performance than total sleep deprivation (short or long term).

People with chronically poor sleep also have more car accidents. And among people with chronic conditions, lack of sleep predicts greater functional disability and decreased quality of life. Not surprisingly, people with poor sleep use more medical services than do their non-sleep-deprived counterparts (Stepanski et al., 2003).

Smith and colleagues (2000) noted the overlap between sleep and pain, with the relationship most likely being bi-directional: pain interferes with sleep and sleep disturbances increase the experience of pain. Sleep problems may also reduce a patient's ability to cope with chronic pain. In their study of 51 people with chronic pain, 88 percent reported some dissatisfaction with their sleep. Pre-sleep cognitive hyperarousal was the best predictor of sleep quality, regardless of pain severity. This included racing thoughts, intrusive thoughts, depressive cognitions, and worry.

The deleterious effects of disturbed sleep have also been found in samples of trauma survivors. In a sample of female rape survivors with posttraumatic stress disorder, trauma-related sleep disorders had an independent impact on health, even after controlling for both depression and PTSD (Clum *et al.*, 2001).

TREATMENT OF SLEEP DISORDERS
The field of sleep medicine can provide us with effective strategies to deal with poor sleep quality. Krakow *et al.* (2000) noted that since sleep medicine is not well integrated into trauma treatment, practitioners are often less effective than they could be if they also treated underlying sleep disorders. They noted that psychotropic medications may mask the presentation of an underlying sleep disorder, meaning that it doesn't get treated. Prescribers may actually exacerbate the psychiatric illness they are striving to treat by prescribing the medication in the first place.

To begin with, practitioners must first assess trauma survivors for possible sleep disorders. In fact, Morin and Ware (1996) recommend that a systematic assessment of sleep be incorporated into all psychological evaluations. They suggest that practitioners ask about the onset of the sleep disorder, and the temporal sequence of when the sleep disorder and the psychiatric disorder manifested. Did the symptoms of the psychiatric disorder pre-date the onset of sleep problems or vice versa?

Polysomnigraphic studies can also reveal whether there are any sleep-breathing or sleep-movement disorders that might also be treated. These conditions often improve with medications and/or assistive devices. However, cognitive-behavioral interventions are appropriate for treating most sleep problems. These techniques are briefly described below.

COGNITIVE-BEHAVIORAL INTERVENTION FOR SLEEP DIFFICULTIES
Cognitive-behavioral intervention has proven effective in the treatment of sleep disorders. In one recent review, it was effective for 70 percent to 80 percent of patients, and was comparable to sleep medications (Morin, 2004; Stepanski and Perlis, 2000). Cognitive-behavioral interventions help with sleep because they produce changes in REM sleep. Cognitive approaches can also address worry and rumination that may be at the base of primary or secondary insomnia (Morin and Ware, 1996).

Cognitive therapy for insomnia includes three components: behavioral, cognitive, and educational. These include establishing regular bedtimes, not using the bed for anything other than sleeping and sex, getting out of bed when unable to sleep, and eliminating naps during the day. There is also a relaxation component that focuses on both autonomic relaxation techniques (e.g., progressive muscle relaxation), and cognitive techniques that stop the worrying that keeps people from sleeping. Cognitive therapy addresses some of the faulty beliefs associated with not sleeping. For example, patients may believe that there are dire consequences of not sleeping. Finally, sleep-hygiene education helps people minimize behaviors that might interfere with sleep. This might include eliminating caffeine, exercise, alcohol, and smoking too close to bedtime (Morin, 2004; Stepanski and Perlis, 2000). A combination of these approaches is effective for most patients with sleep disorders.

CONCLUSION
Sleep disorders are another common effect of trauma that can increase health problems in trauma survivors. By recognizing possible sleep disorders, practitioners can help patients minimize, or even eliminate, sleep problems. This will likely result in lower levels of symptoms and improved health overall.

IMPLICATIONS

The research literature in health psychology and behavioral medicine has identified two areas where intervention is likely to have a substantial impact on the health of trauma survivors. These interventions would improve self-efficacy and quality of sleep. Although these are not currently part of standard trauma treatment, or even standard primary care, a large body of research indicates that these would be fruitful areas to explore. By improving patients' self-efficacy, we give them tools to help themselves. And by improving patients' sleep quality, we would likely decrease their trauma symptoms and increase their ability to cope because they just feel better. In either case, patients would improve and their treatment would be more effective. It's worth a closer look even though it's "thinking outside the box."

REFERENCES

Alewijnse, D., Mesters, I, Metsemakers, J., Adrianns, J., and van den Borne, B. (2001). Predictors of intention to adhere to physiotherapy among women with urinary incontinence. *Health Education Research, 16,* 173–186.

Bandura, A. (1999). A sociocognitive analysis of substance abuse: An agentic perspective. *Psychological Science, 10,* 214–217.

Bray, S.R., and Cowan, H. (2004). Proxy efficacy: Implications for self-efficacy and exercise intentions in cardiac rehabilitation. *Rehabilitation Psychology, 49,* 71–75.

Brown, L.K., Kessel, S.M., Lourie, K.J., and Ford, H.H. (1997). Influence of sexual abuse on HIV-related attitudes and behaviors in adolescent psychiatric inpatients. *Journal of the American Academy of Child and Adolescent Psychiatry, 36,* 316–322.

Brown, L.K., Lourie, K.J., Zlotnick, C., and Cohn, J. (2000). Impact of sexual abuse on the HIV-risk-related behavior of adolescents in intensive psychiatric treatment. *American Journal of Psychiatry, 157,* 1413–1415.

Carmichael, C.L., and Reis, H.T. (2005). Attachment, sleep quality, and depressed affect. *Health Psychology, 24,* 526–531.

Catz, S.L., Kelly, J.A., Bogard, L.M., Benotsch, E.G., and McAuliffe, T.L. (2000). Patterns, correlates, and barriers to medication adherence among persons prescribed new treatments for HIV disease. *Health Psychology, 19,* 124–133.

Chambers, E., and Belicki, K. (1998). Using sleep dysfunction to explore the nature of resilience in adult survivors of childhood abuse or trauma. *Child Abuse and Neglect, 22*, 753–758.

Choquet, M., Darves-Bornoz, J-M., Ledoux, S., Manfredi, R., and Hassler, C. (1997). Self-reported health and behavioral problems among adolescent victims of rape in France: Results of a cross-sectional survey. *Child Abuse and Neglect, 21*, 823–832.

Clum, G.A., Nishith, P., and Resick, P.A. (2001). Trauma-related sleep disturbance and self-reported physical health symptoms in treatment-seeking female rape victims. *Journal of Nervous and Mental Disease, 189*, 618–622.

Dobkin, P.L., Abrahamowicz, M., Fitzcharles, M-A., Dritsa, M., and daCosta, D. (2005). Maintenance of exercise in women with fibromyalgia. *Arthritis Care and Research, 53*, 724–731.

Franko, D.L., Streigel-Moore, R.H., Bean, J., Tamer, R., Kraemer, H.C., *et al.* (2005). Psychosocial and health consequences of adolescent depression in Black and White young adult women. *Health Psychology, 24*, 586–593.

Fuller, K.H., Waters, W.F., Binks, P.G., and Anderson, T. (1997). Generalized anxiety and sleep architecture: A polysomnographic investigation. *Sleep, 20*, 370–376.

Heinrichs, M., Wagner, D., Schoch, W., Soravia, L.M., Hellhammer, D.H., and Ehlert, U. (2005). Predicting posttraumatic stress symptoms from pretraumatic risk factors: A 2-year prospective follow-up study in firefighters. *American Journal of Psychiatry, 162*, 2276–2286.

Hulme, P.A. (2000). Symptomatology and health care utilization of women primary care patients who experienced childhood sexual abuse. *Child Abuse and Neglect, 24*, 1471–1484.

Humphreys, J.C., Lee, K.A., Neylan, T.C., and Marmar, C.R. (1999). Sleep patterns of sheltered battered women. *Journal of Nursing Scholarship, 31*, 139–143.

Jones, K.D., Burckhardt, C.S., and Bennett, J.A. (2004). Motivational interviewing may encourage exercise in persons with fibromyalgia by enhancing self-efficacy. *Arthritis Care and Research, 51*, 864–867.

Jump, R.L., Fifield, J., Tennen, H., Reisine, S., and Giullano, A.J. (2004). History of affective disorder and the experience of fatigue in rheumatoid arthritis. *Arthritis Care and Research, 51*, 239–245.

Kaplan, R.M., Ries, A.L., Prewitt, L.A., and Eakin, E. (1994). Self-efficacy expectations predict survival for patients with chronic obstructive pulmonary disease. *Health Psychology, 13*, 366–368.

Koss, M.P. (1990). The women's mental health research agenda: Violence against women. *American Psychologist, 45*, 374–380.

Krakow, B., Artar, A., Warner, T.D., Melendez, D., Johnston, L., Hollifield, M., Gemain, A., and Koss, M. (2000). Sleep disorder, depression, and suicidality in female sexual assault survivors. *Crisis, 21*, 163–170.

Langenberg, P., Ballesteros, M., Feldman, R., Damron, D., Anliker, J., and Havas, S. (2000). Psychosocial factors and intervention-associated changes in those factors as correlates of change in fruit and vegetable consumption in the Maryland WIC 5 a Day promotion program. *Annals of Behavioral Medicine, 22*, 307–315.

Leserman, J., Li, Z., Drossman, D.A., and Hu, Y.J.B. (1998). Selected symptoms associated with sexual and physical abuse history among female patients with gastrointestinal disorders: The impact on subsequent health care visits. *Psychological Medicine, 28*, 417–425.

Macrodimitris, S.D., and Endler, N.S. (2001). Coping, control, and adjustment in Type 2 diabetes. *Health Psychology, 20*, 208–216.

Mahler, H.I.M., and Kulik, J.A. (1998). Effects of preparatory videotapes on self-efficacy beliefs and recovery from coronary bypass surgery. *Annals of Behavioral Medicine, 20*, 39–46.

Mann, T. (2001). Effects of future writing and optimism on health behaviors in HIV-infected women. *Annals of Behavioral Medicine, 23*, 26–33.

Marks, R. (2001). Efficacy theory and its utility in arthritis rehabilitation: Review and recommendations. *Disability and Rehabilitation: An International Multidisciplinary Journal, 23*, 271–280.

McAuley, E., Blissmer, B., Katula, J., Duncan, T.E., and Mihalko, S.L. (2000). Physical activity, self-esteem, and self-efficacy relationships in older adults: A randomized controlled trial. *Annals of Behavioral Medicine, 22*, 131–139.

McAuley, E., and Courneya, K.S. (1993). Adherence to exercise and physical activity as health-promoting behaviors: Attitudinal and self-efficacy influences. *Applied and Preventive Psychology, 2*, 65–77.

Mohr, D.C., Boudewyn, A.C., Likosky, W., Levine, E., and Goodkin, D.E. (2001). Injectable medication for the treatment of multiple sclerosis: The influence of self-efficacy expectations and injection anxiety on adherence and ability to self-inject. *Annals of Behavioral Medicine, 23*, 125–132.

Moos, R.H., and Cronkite, R.C. (1999). Symptom-based predictors of a 10-year chronic course of treated depression. *Journal of Nervous and Mental Disease, 187*, 360–368.

Morin, C.M. (2004). Cognitive-behavioral approaches to the treatment of insomnia. *Journal of Clinical Psychiatry, 65 [suppl]*, 33–40.

Morin, C.M., and Ware, J.C. (1996). Sleep and psychopathology. *Applied and Preventive Psychology, 5*, 211–224.

Nicassio, P.M., and Wallston, K.A. (1992). Longitudinal relationships among pain, sleep problems, and depression in rheumatoid arthritis. *Journal of Abnormal Psychology, 101*, 514–520.

Norman, P., Bennett, P., Smith, C., and Murphy, S. (1998). Health locus of control and health behavior. *Journal of Health Psychology, 3*, 171–180.

Oliver, J.M., and Paull, J.C. (1995). Self-esteem and self-efficacy; perceived parenting and family climate; and depression in university students. *Journal of Clinical Psychology, 51*, 467–481.

Orbell, S., Johnston, M., Rowley, D., Davey, P., and Espley, A. (2001). Self-efficacy and goal importance in the prediction of physical disability in people following hospitalization: A prospective study. *British Journal of Health Psychology, 6*, 25–41.

Perlis, M.L., Giles, D.E., Buysse, D.J., Thase, M.E., Tu, X., and Kupfer, D.J. (1997). Which depressive symptoms are related to which sleep electroencephalographic variables? *Biological Psychiatry, 42*, 904–913.

Pilcher, J.J., and Huffcutt, A.I. (1996). Effects of sleep deprivation on performance: A meta-analysis. *Sleep, 19*, 318–326.

Roberts, R.E., Shema, S.J., Kaplan, G.A., and Strawbridge, W.J. (2000). Sleep complaints and depression in an aging cohort: A prospective perspective. *American Journal of Psychiatry, 157*, 81–88.

Ryan, N.E., Solberg, V.S., and Brown, S.D. (1996). Family dysfunction, parental attachment, and career search self-efficacy among community college students. *Journal of Counseling Psychology, 43*, 84–89.

Sacco, W.P., Wells, K.J., Vaughan, C.A., Friedman, A., Perez, S., and Matthew, R. (2005). Depression in adults with type 2 diabetes: The role of adherence, body mass index, and self-efficacy. *Health Psychology, 24*, 630–634.

Sanz, A., and Villamarin, F. (2001). The role of perceived control in physiological reactivity: Self-efficacy and incentive value as regulators of cardiovascular adjustment. *Biological Psychology, 56*, 219–246.

Siegel, K., Schrimshaw, E.W., and Dean, L. (1999). Symptom interpretation and medication adherence among late middle-age and older HIV-infected adults. *Journal of Health Psychology, 4*, 247–257.

Simoni, J.M., Frick, P.A., and Huang, B. (2006). A longitudinal evaluation of a social support model of medication adherence among HIV-positive men and women on antiretroviral therapy. *Health Psychology, 25*, 74–81.

Smith, M.T., Perlis, M.L., Smith, M.S., Giles, D.E., and Carmody, T.P. (2000). Sleep quality and presleep arousal in chronic pain. *Journal of Behavioral Medicine, 23*, 1–13.

Smyth, J.M., Stone, A.A., Hurewitz, A., and Kaell, A. (1999). Effects of writing about stressful experiences on symptom reduction in patients with asthma or rheumatoid arthritis. *Journal of the American Medical Association, 281*, 1304–1309.

Stepanski, E.J., and Perlis, M.L. (2000). Behavioral sleep medicine: An emerging subspecialty in health psychology and sleep medicine. *Journal of Psychosomatic Research, 49*, 343–347.

Stepanski, E.J., Rybarczyk, B., Lopez, M., and Stevens, S. (2003). Assessment and treatment of sleep disorders in older adults: A review for rehabilitation psychologists. *Rehabilitation Psychology, 48*, 23–36.

Teegen, F. (1999). Childhood sexual abuse and long-term sequelae. In A. Maercker, M. Schutzwohl, and Z. Solomon (eds), *Posttraumatic stress disorder: A lifespan developmental perspective* (pp. 97–112). Seattle: Hogrefe & Huber.

Torres, J.B., and Solberg, V.S. (2001). Role of self-efficacy, stress, social integration, and family support in Latino college student persistence and health. *Journal of Vocational Behavior, 59*, 53–63.

Toth, S.L., and Cicchetti, D. (1996). Patterns of relatedness, depressive symptomatology, and perceived competence in maltreated children. *Journal of Consulting and Clinical Psychology, 64*, 32–41.

Waldrop, D., Lightsey, O.R., Ethington, C.A., Woemmel, C.A., and Coke, A.L. (2001). Self-efficacy, optimism, health competence, and recovery from orthopedic surgery. *Journal of Counseling Psychology, 48*, 233–238.

Wallston, K.A. (2001). Conceptualization and operationalization of perceived control. In A. Baum, T.A. Revenson, and J.E. Singer (eds), *Handbook of health psychology* (pp. 49–58). Mahwah, NJ: Lawrence Erlbaum.

Walsh, J.F., and Foshee, V. (1998). Self-efficacy, self-determination and victim blaming as predictors of adolescent sexual victimization. *Health Education Research, 13*, 139–144.

Ware, J.C., and Morin, C.M. (1997). Sleep in depression and anxiety. In M.R. Pressman and W.C. Orr (eds), *Understanding sleep: The evaluation and treatment of sleep disorders* (pp. 483–503). Washington, DC: American Psychological Association.

Weinberg, N.S., Sroufe, L.A., Egeland, B., and Carlson, E.A. (1999). The nature of individual differences in infant-caregiver attachment. In J. Cassidy and P.R. Shaver (eds), *The handbook of attachment: Theory, research, and clinical applications* (pp. 68–88). New York: Guilford Press.

Where does it hurt?

How victimization impacts presentation and outcomes in primary care

Stephanie Dallam

"If somebody discloses [sexual abuse] for the first time
. . . to me, it's like a Pandora's box and I just wouldn't
know what to do. I wouldn't know what to do with this
stuff coming out."

Nurse in community-based clinic
(quoted by Tudiver *et al.*, 2000, p. 23)

IN AN EFFORT TO PROVIDE appropriate care, the importance of
a thorough health history is widely recognized. However, many
practitioners fail to recognize the importance a history of
victimization can have on subsequent health outcomes. Thus,
while health care providers routinely ask about prior surgeries,
illnesses, and broken bones, few ask about exposure to violence
or experiences of victimization. Increased recognition of the
long-term impact of victimization on patients' health has led to a
call for integrating assessment for victimization into routine care
(e.g., American Medical Association, 1995; Family Violence
Prevention Fund, 2004).

The purpose of this chapter is to provide an overview of why
a victimization history can be an important consideration during

all phases of the health care encounter. Identification of trauma-related problems in primary care settings can not only improve diagnosis and treatment, it can also improve patient satisfaction and compliance.

PREVALENCE OF VICTIMIZATION IN PRIMARY CARE

Child maltreatment occurs at epidemic numbers. A recent random national survey of the United States adult population revealed that 14 percent of men and 32 percent of women reported childhood experiences that satisfied criteria for sexual abuse (Briere and Elliott, 2003). Twenty-one percent of those who experienced sexual abuse had also experienced physical abuse, and both types of abuse were associated with subsequent victimization as an adult. Domestic violence and adult sexual assaults are also highly prevalent in our society. Using a nationally representative sample, the Commonwealth Fund's 1998 Survey of Women's Health found that 20.4 percent of women are likely to experience rape during their lifetime, and 34.6 percent to experience intimate partner violence (Plichta and Falik, 2001).

The rate of a victimization history in health care settings may be even higher, as victimization is associated with increased complaints that result in survivors being disproportionately frequent users of health care services (Bohn and Holz, 1996; Plichta and Falik, 2001). A study of 557 women in a primary care setting found that over 70 percent of the women had experienced physical, emotional, and/or sexual abuse at some point in their lives (Carlson *et al.*, 2003). Unfortunately, most health care providers are unaware of their client's abuse history because health care providers rarely ask and most patients do not volunteer this information (McCauley *et al.*, 1998).

The unspoken policy in most health care settings appears to be one of "don't ask, don't tell." A cross-sectional survey of over 2,000 women seen by general practitioners found that few patients disclosed this fact to their doctor. An abuse history was revealed by only 27 percent of those who had experienced partner violence, 27 percent who experienced childhood physical abuse, and 9 percent of those who had experienced sexual abuse (Mazza *et al.*, 1996). Similar rates were reported by Plichta and Falik (2001) in their Survey of Women's Health; only one-third of women who experienced violence had discussed it with a physician. It appears that many patients fail to disclose an abuse history because their provider has never raised the subject.

A study of 162 women attending a primary care clinic found that 37 percent had experienced childhood sexual abuse and 29 percent had experienced adult sexual assault. Although most of the women believed it was appropriate for their physician to ask about previous victimization, only 4 percent had been asked (Walker *et al.*, 1993).

HEALTH OUTCOMES

Many practitioners fail to ask about victimization because they fail to see the relevance of past traumatic experiences to current symptomology. Research, however, implicates a victimization history as a risk factor in a number of debilitating psychiatric conditions and with poorer physical health throughout the lifespan. For instance, chronically traumatized children may display signs of posttraumatic stress disorder (PTSD), attention deficit hyperactivity disorder (ADHD), major depression, various dissociative disorders, oppositional-defiant disorder, conduct disorder, separation anxiety, or specific phobia (Perry and Azad, 1999; Perry *et al.*, 1995).

Childhood victimization is similarly correlated with a wide range of psychiatric disorders in adulthood including depression, PTSD, panic disorder, dissociation, and somatization (Briere and Runtz, 1988; Kendler *et al.*, 2000; Molnar *et al.*, 2001; Morse *et al.*, 1997). A history of victimization is similarly associated with numerous health problems during adulthood. The effects of maltreatment on adult physical health may be divided into three overlapping categories: (1) health care utilization; (2) subjective health perceptions, physical complaints, and functional disorders; and (3) occurrence of serious illness and chronic disease.

HEATH CARE UTILIZATION

A history of physical or sexual assault during either childhood or adulthood has been found to be a powerful predictor of subsequent increased health care utilization (Bergman and Brismar, 1991; Felitti, 1991; Koss et al., 1990; Tang et al., in press). For example, research has shown that abused women use a disproportionate amount of health care services, including primary care medical visits, emergency room visits, community mental health center visits, and prescriptions (Farley and Patsalides, 2001; Plichta, 1992). Abused woman also tend to be admitted to hospital more frequently and undergo more surgical procedures than their non-abused peers (Moeller et al., 1993; Salmon and Calderbank, 1996).

HEALTH PERCEPTIONS, PHYSICAL COMPLAINTS, AND FUNCTIONAL DISORDERS

A history of childhood maltreatment is significantly associated with lower self-ratings of overall health, with those experiencing multiple types of maltreatment reporting the worst health (Golding et al., 1997; Walker et al., 1999a, 1999b). A strong, graded relationship has also been found between severity of past victimization and physical complaints in adulthood (Golding et al., 1997; Moeller et al., 1993). A study of women found that recent as well as past victimization was associated with poorer health status including more pain, symptoms, bed disability days, physician visits, functional disability, and psychological distress (Leserman et al., 1998). Childhood maltreatment is strongly associated with unexplained medical complaints, with abused women reporting problems in twice as many body systems as non-abused women (Lechner et al., 1993).

A childhood maltreatment history appears to be a risk factor for a wide variety of functional health problems. A disease is considered "functional" when no organic cause can be found to explain a patient's somatic complaints. A history of victimization has been found to be associated with the following functional disorders: chronic pelvic pain (Drossman et al., 1990;

Harrop-Griffiths *et al.*, 1988; Heim *et al.*, 1998; Reiter *et al.*, 1991; Springs and Friedrich, 1992), irritable bowel syndrome (Drossman *et al.*, 1990), fibromyalgia (Boisset-Pioro *et al.*, 1995; Imbierowicz and Egle, 2003), musculoskeletal pain (Drossman *et al.*, 1990; Leserman *et al.*, 1998; Linton, 1997), premenstrual dysphoric disorder (Girdler *et al.*, 1998, 2003), chronic headaches (Domino and Haber, 1987; Drossman *et al.*, 1990; Felitti, 1991; Romans *et al.*, 2002), and chronic fatigue (Drossman *et al.*, 1990; Romans *et al.*, 2002). Many of these disorders are co-occurring. For instance, about half of women with chronic pelvic pain also have irritable bowel syndrome (Whitehead *et al.*, 2002); and women with fibromyalgia frequently suffer from numerous other unexplained disorders including chronic fatigue syndrome, irritable bowel syndrome, temporomandibular disorder, and chronic headaches (Aaron and Buchwald, 2001).

SERIOUS ILLNESS AND CHRONIC DISEASE
A history of victimization is associated with increased rates of serious illness and chronic disease. For instance, data from a nationally representative sample containing over 5,000 adults revealed that childhood maltreatment was associated with a significant increase in cardiovascular disease for women (Batten *et al.*, 2004). A random survey found that a number of illnesses were reported more often in women who had experienced various forms of sexual and physical abuse, both in childhood and in adult life. These included chronic fatigue, bladder problems, headaches, asthma, diabetes, and heart problems (Romans *et al.*, 2002). Associations have also been found between early sexual abuse and several health conditions in the elderly. Stein and Barrett-Connor (2000) analyzed health data on more than 1,300 elderly white, middle-class men and women from a southern California community. In women, early sexual assault appeared to increase the risk of arthritis and breast cancer, with multiple abuse episodes increasing disease risk by two- to three-fold compared with a single episode. In men, early sexual assault appeared to increase the risk of thyroid disease.

The most comprehensive study of the effects of childhood maltreatment on adult health is the Adverse Childhood Experiences (ACE) Study. The ACE Study is a large-scale, ongoing epidemiological study that assesses the impact of numerous adverse childhood experiences on a variety of health behaviors and outcomes in adulthood. The investigators surveyed over 17,000 adults on adverse childhood experiences soon after they had a standardized medical evaluation at a large health maintenance organization (HMO). The participants were questioned about the presence of eight, then ten, adverse experiences during childhood including psychological, physical, or sexual abuse; violence against the mother; or living with household members who were substance abusers, mentally ill or suicidal, or ever imprisoned. The results revealed a strong, graded relationship between the number of categories of adverse experiences and the presence of serious adult diseases including ischemic heart disease, cancer, chronic lung disease, skeletal fractures, and liver disease. For example, those who experienced four or more categories of adverse childhood experiences were 60 percent more likely to have diabetes, twice as likely to suffer cancer, stroke, or heart disease (Felitti *et al.*, 1998). Taken together, these findings suggest that childhood maltreatment and household dysfunction may be related to the development of chronic diseases that are among the most common causes of death and disability in the United States.

THE MEDIATING EFFECT OF PSYCHOLOGICAL DISTRESS AND HEALTH-RISK BEHAVIORS

Although the specific pathways through which victimization may be related to adult health are unknown, various neurobiological and behavioral responses to the stress of victimization may provide the framework through which early abuse is transformed from psychosocial experience into both mental illness and organic disease (Anda *et al.*, 2006; Felitti, 2002). Increasingly sophisticated neurobiological studies show that early trauma may adversely influence brain development and permanently alter the functioning of biological stress response systems including the hypothalamic–pituitary–adrenal (HPA) axis. After an episode of acute stress, feedback mechanisms turn off the stress-response, returning the system to baseline. However, when trauma is severe and ongoing, compensatory mechanisms may become over-activated and incapable of restoring the brain's previous state of equilibrium. The physiological system is then forced to reorganize its basal patterns. The more intense and prolonged the traumatic event, the more likely there will be reorganization of these neural systems. This reorganization of the neural systems can lead to sensitization of the HPA axis rendering the body increasingly reactive to stress (De Bellis, 2002; Penza et al., 2003; Teicher, 2002).

There is increasing evidence that disorders which have been considered "functional" may in fact result from HPA axis dysfunction similar to that found in PTSD and depression (Dallam, 2001, 2005; Heim et al., 1998; Kendall-Tackett, 2003). HPA dysfunction is associated with functional conditions such as fibromyalgia, irritable bowel syndrome, somatization, and chronic pain syndromes (Crofford, 1996; Gracely et al., 2002; Gutman and Nemeroff, 2003; Heim et al., 1998; Milla, 2001). Chronic stress has also been shown to affect immune functioning. For instance, prolonged periods of stress are associated with high levels of the proinflammatory cytokine, interleukin-6 (IL-6). High IL-6 levels are associated with cardiovascular disease, depression, osteoporosis, arthritis, Type-2 diabetes, and some cancers (Kiecolt-Glaser et al., 2003).

The relationship between victimization and health may be further mediated by behavioral reactions to abuse. Numerous studies have found a history of victimization to be associated with higher rates of a wide variety of health risk behaviors (Diaz et al., 2000; Felitti et al., 1998; Fergusson et al., 1997; Raj et al., 2000). Many of these behaviors have been identified by the Centers for Disease Control (2003) as contributing dramatically to leading causes of morbidity and mortality in adults including cardiovascular disease, diabetes, and cancer. For instance, in its survey of mostly middle-aged adult HMO members, the ACE Study found a strong graded relationship between the numbers of different adversities experienced in childhood and *every* health risk behavior studied, including cigarette smoking, obesity, physical inactivity, alcoholism, drug abuse, depression, suicide attempts, sexual promiscuity, and sexually transmitted diseases. Many of these relationships were quite strong. For example, those who experienced four or more types of adverse childhood experiences were more than seven times more likely to consider themselves to be an alcoholic, almost five times more likely to have used illicit drugs, and more than ten times more likely to have injected illicit drugs (Felitti *et al.*, 1998). Further analysis revealed that adverse events during childhood may account for one-half to two-thirds of serious problems with drug use (Dube *et al.*, 2003).

Although the pathways between victimization and participation in risky behaviors have yet to be elucidated, engaging in health risk behaviors may reflect an attempt to regulate stress-related changes in brain chemistry (Anda *et al.*, 2006). Evidence of a causal relationship between victimization and use of mood-altering substances is provided by a longitudinal study of a national probability sample of 3,006 women. Investigators found that after a new sexual assault, odds of both alcohol abuse and drug usage were significantly increased, even among women with no previous substance use or assault history (Kilpatrick *et al.*, 1997). Further support for a causal relationship is provided by numerous clinical studies in which addicted women have reported using substances expressly for the purpose of coping with the adverse effects of victimization (Ballon *et al.*, 2001; Harrison *et al.*, 1989).

HOW VICTIMIZATION CAN AFFECT THE QUALITY OF HEALTH CARE ENCOUNTERS

In addition to its effect on mental and physical health, a history of victimization can also influence the quality of health care encounters in a number of important ways. First, it can influence patients' relationships with their bodies and their response to somatic symptoms. Second, because health care settings and situations often contain potent reminders of abuse, patients with a history of victimization may experience debilitating posttraumatic reactions during health care encounters. A final means through which victimization can affect the health care encounter is by influencing patients' sense of safety and trust when in the care of others.

THE PATIENT'S RELATIONSHIP WITH THEIR BODY

A history of abuse can negatively impact patients' relationships with their bodies and impair their ability to interpret somatic symptoms. In a study of abuse survivors with somatization, the women interviewed described having low self-esteem and difficulty discerning the meaning of symptoms (Morse *et al.*, 1997). Growing up, their feelings and their pain did not matter to their parents, creating a sense of distrust for what they felt. One survivor noted,

> **It's not having bad things happen, it's that there is just nobody every place you turn that will tell you it's true and it's really awful. If you're angry and you're told you're not; if you're hurt, you're not; if you're sad, you're not. How can you believe anything you feel?**
>
> **(Morse *et al.*, 1997, p. 473)**

Abuse survivors may feel that their bodies have been deformed or ruined by abuse. Those who have experienced sexual assaults may consider their bodies disgusting because they attracted the abuser or feel betrayed by their bodies because they responded to someone's touch (Kitzinger, 1992). Some survivors blame themselves for the abuse rather than the perpetrator, and as a result view themselves as deserving of abuse and unworthy of care. Abuse survivors may cut or burn their bodies as a form of "self-punishment" or to cope with painful emotions (Dallam, 1997; Haas and Popp, 2006). This estrangement from the body can make it more difficult for survivors to recognize when to seek medical attention, and may render them less likely to follow through with recommendations to improve their health.

RETRAUMATIZATION

A second means by which a victimization history can influence the quality of health care encounters is through their potential for retraumatization. Retraumatization in health care settings refers to the triggering of posttraumatic symptoms in response to situations within the health care environment that are reminiscent of prior traumas for patients seeking care. As a result the trauma survivor may experience cognitive, emotional, and physical reactions that are more appropriate for the original trauma than for the present situation. Retraumatization appears to have its roots in posttraumatic symptoms such as those found in PTSD. A common response to victimization, PTSD is a syndrome that involves symptoms of intrusive re-experiencing of the trauma, avoidance and/or emotional numbing, and autonomic hyperarousal (American Psychiatric Association, 1994). Research suggests that the lifetime prevalence of PTSD among survivors of physical and sexual assault is about 31 percent, which is similar to the prevalence reported for combat exposure (Ford et al., 1996). Part of the psychological response to trauma involves oscillation between avoidance of the event's emotional impact and re-experiencing distress when exposed to reminders of the trauma (Horowitz, 1986).

Interviews with abuse survivors suggest that health care settings are replete with reminders for victims of interpersonal violence (Kitzinger, 1992; Schachter et al., 1999; Seng et al., 2002; Stalker et al., 2005). A study of 39 survivors of childhood sexual abuse found that over half were reminded of sexual assaults by their visits to doctors or dentists (Kitzinger, 1992). Medical procedures that involve physical contact with previously traumatized areas of the body (such as the mouth, neck, breasts, genitals, and rectum) or involve inserting objects into the body can recapitulate aspects of the assault (American Medical Association, 1995; see Table 6.1).

TABLE 6.1 Medical situations which may cause re-experiencing of trauma

Procedures that involve previously traumatized areas of the body (e.g., the mouth, neck, breasts, genitals, and rectum)

Procedures that require disrobing

Inadequate privacy arrangements

Procedures that occur in a darkened room (such as an eye exam)

Procedures that require being confined to a small place (MRI, CT scan)

Procedures that restrict the patient's mobility (e.g., MRI, CT scan, restraints)

Procedures in which objects are inserted into the body (e.g., catheters, needles, endoscopic procedures)

Medications that affect mental alertness or functioning (such as anesthesia)

Open discord between care staff members

Loud noises

Practitioner resembles the patient's abuser in some way

Source: Adapted from American Medical Association (1995)

The vulnerability that comes with being a patient may also be a source of much distress. Schachter *et al.* (1999) interviewed 27 female survivors of childhood abuse who had received physical therapy or who had considered seeing a physical therapist upon referral. Recalling having to put on a paper gown, one survivor stated, "The first time I went there and I had to wear this thing, I felt so exposed and so naked and, and hated it" (Schachter *et al.*, 1999, p. 257). The vulnerability of being placed in laying or sitting positions during procedures may also lead to not feeling safe. A male survivor of child sexual abuse described his difficulty going to the dentist: "I just get that feeling . . . when you have no control because you're in the chair, your mouth is frozen, and you're pretty much at the mercy of that person" (Stalker *et al.*, 2005, p. 1277).

Uncertainty about what was happening around them can also lead to safety concerns. In describing medical personnel busily going about their business around her, one woman stated, "That's when I get really uncomfortable and I tense up. And I want to push them away, and I want to run, leave" (Schachter *et al.*, 1999, p. 255). A survivor in physical therapy noted that the element of surprise was really difficult to deal with because she never knew when "I will be triggered by something that is done, you know, into remembering something that is abusive for me" (Schachter *et al.*, 1999, p. 255).

Some survivors have difficulty tolerating physical touch. Schachter *et al.* (1999) found that some survivors are able to tolerate touch in some areas of their body but not in others; while others found it difficult regardless of where they were touched. Items that are routinely used in providing care can also act as triggers for some patients. For example, a physical therapy patient with a history of childhood sexual abuse reported reactivation of trauma symptoms due to the gel used during ultrasound treatments. She stated, "the goop that they put on me for the ultrasound gave me flashbacks, nightmares, insomnia. I just couldn't deal with it" (Schachter *et al.*, 1999, p. 257). Another sexual abuse survivor reported difficulty with procedures requiring the use of latex gloves, noting that "the gloves smell like condoms" (Stalker *et al.*, 2005, p. 1281).

REACTIONS AND COPING

When faced with situations or procedures reminiscent of abuse, many survivors of childhood abuse respond by using the same types of coping mechanisms they utilized as a child. One of the main coping mechanisms reported is dissociation, which tends to shut down emotions before they occur outwardly. Dissociation is defined as constituting "a structured separation of mental processes (e.g., thoughts, emotions, conation, memory, and identity) that are normally integrated" (Spiegel and Cardena, 1991, p. 366). According to Perry (2000), the normal response to danger – to fight or flee – is usually unfeasible for a small child.

Therefore, traumatized children frequently use a "freeze" or surrender response in which the child dissociates from the events around her and withdraws inwardly. Dissociation allows the child to distance themselves from overwhelming emotional or physical pain, while at the same remaining compliant with the demands of the abuser. An abuse survivor interviewed by Schachter *et al.* (1999, p. 254) described how she reacted to an event during physical therapy that upset her.

> **I really freaked but . . . I didn't show her I was freaking, because our history is that, you don't let on if things are a problem for you. You just deal with it however you can . . . by dissociating or what have you.**

Overall, Schachter *et al.* (1999) found that when distressed, abuse survivors tended to acquiesce, while weakly communicating their disagreement through passive non-verbal signals and dissociation. Survivors who coped by dissociating often reported having difficulty remembering what the provider had told them during their visit. Abuse survivors interviewed by Seng *et al.* (2002) described similar reactions. One woman described how the dissociative defenses she used to cope with the abuse were automatically reactivated in maternity care. She stated, "my reactions to pregnancy, becoming submissive again . . . I was completely passive . . . I didn't advocate for myself at all." She attributed her response to a lack of control, and someone else in authority "calling the shots no matter what I really wanted" (p. 367). She reported later not remembering "what exactly went on" (p. 367).

Most abuse survivors recognize that some of their reactions are not consistent with the current situation and are embarrassed and frustrated both by their reactions and the inability of health care providers to understand them. One survivor had come to recognize her triggers and would tell her physical therapists what she could handle that day. She felt the need for her wishes to be respected without being "treated like some sort of baby . . . or . . . 'What's your problem?' kind of thing" (p. 254). In a firsthand account, another sexual abuse survivor noted her embarrassment over her reactions to dental situations. She said that she frequently worried during dental situations that she might lose it and "behave like a frightened small child" and expressed concern over what her dentist and nurse would then think of her. She noted that at times she had "wished the ground would open up and swallow me," and felt that she could never go back (Anonymous, 2004).

To cope with their feelings of increased vulnerability, abuse survivors interviewed by Schachter et al. (1999) frequently described their need for a sense of control over what happens to them during health care procedures. A survivor in physical therapy noted, "[B]eing a survivor. I have to be in charge, I guess, and if I'm not in charge. . . . It's an awful feeling" p. 255).

PATIENTS' TRUST IN AND EXPECTATIONS OF THE PROVIDER
A final means through which victimization can affect the health care encounter is by affecting patients' ability to trust their provider or feel safe while in his or her care. A study of female survivors of childhood sexual abuse revealed that many feared being abused during health care visits; and some felt unsafe working with male health care providers (Schachter et al., 1999). A study by McNutt and colleagues (2000) examined the relationship between victimization by an intimate partner and patient satisfaction with medical encounters among African-American woman. Victimized women were less likely to report that they felt respected and accepted during the encounter, and they provided lower ratings of the quality of communication with their providers.

Another study found a general association between lifetime experiences of emotional, physical, and/or sexual abuse and perceived abuse in the health care system (Swahnberg et al., 2004). For some patients, a distrust of medical providers may date back to childhood. A study of sexual abuse victims with somatization found that many had childhood physicians who were family members or the abuser's physician, which reinforced subsequent distrust of medical personnel and secrecy about the abuse (Morse *et al.*, 1997).

When one understands the core harm of child abuse, it is no mystery why a history of victimization can negatively impact patients' relationships with health care providers. Child abuse typically occurs at the hands of a trusted caretaker and thus challenges deeply held assumptions of safety, fairness, ability to control events, and predictability. Trust, which has been recognized as a key element in therapeutic relationships (Hall *et al.*, 2002), may be difficult for patients who as children were betrayed by those who were supposed to care for them (Courtois, 1988). The experience of being helpless in the hands of an authority figure can recall the powerlessness experienced during abuse. Consequently, for patients who have been harmed by those who were supposed to care for them, relationships with health care providers may be experienced as potentially exploitative situations, which in some cases trigger posttraumatic symptoms (American Medical Association, 1995; Courtois and Riley, 1992; Kitzinger, 1992). Nor does the provider have to behave in a threatening manner for survivors to feel unsafe. Abuse survivors interviewed by Schachter *et al.* (1999) tended to not feel safe when a provider seemed disinterested or rushed. Similar findings were reported by Seng *et al.* (2002) in interviews with abuse survivors regarding childbirth experiences. One survivor said she unexpectedly found herself triggered by the remoteness of the physician providing her prenatal care.

> [T]he doctor was kind of cold, not personable at all, and those feelings [emotional memory of being abused, shame, vulnerability, nakedness] would come back to me in his office, and I found myself crying at every visit.
>
> (Seng *et al.*, 2002, p. 367)

When patients do not trust or feel safe with their provider, they are unlikely to follow through with recommended treatment and follow-up. In interviews with sexual abuse survivors undergoing physical therapy treatment, the women spoke about how their perceived lack of control compromised their feeling of safety and interfered with treatment adherence (Schacter *et al.*, 2004). Anxiety regarding upcoming procedures can also lead patients to cancel appointments and avoid necessary care (Stalker *et al.*, 2005). In other cases, survivors may overuse medical resources by going to multiple specialists trying to find the source of their distressing symptoms. These patients may receive unnecessary and invasive tests, and then experience reactions similar to those experienced as a child when there is lack of confirmation of their suffering (Morse *et al.*, 1997). Some abuse victims may even enjoy the sick role because, as children, they found the medical community to be a source of comfort and safety (Morse *et al.*, 1997). Overall, it seems that for many survivors, relationships with health care providers are difficult, mixed with both hope and dread. Hope that they can be helped; and dread that their concerns will not be taken seriously and their pain discounted. As a result, the provider relationship can unwittingly act as a devastating re-enactment of interpersonal trauma in which the abuse survivor is again left alone to deal with his or her pain.

INCORPORATING AWARENESS OF VICTIMIZATION IN PRACTICE

Improving health outcomes for abuse survivors starts with a victimization history. The literature lists some behavioral "red flags" that should increase suspicion that the patient may have a history of victimization (Table 6.2). Inquiring about abuse can be woven into the health history. The history should be taken with the patient clothed and prior to any procedures. Although it is usually desirable to ensure privacy by closing the door and asking family members to leave when a history is taken, the patient's preferences in this regard should be respected. Some survivors may feel uncomfortable with the examination room door fully clcosed or without the presence of a trusted family member or friend. Guidelines issued by the Florida Council Against Sexual Violence (2002) suggest that providers explain that they are

TABLE 6.2 "Red flags" that should increase suspicion of a victimization history

Poor self-esteem

Addictions

History of chronic depression and/or anxiety attacks

History of PTSD

Eating disorders

Self-destructive behaviors

Sexual dysfunction

History of somatization or functional disorders

Difficulty tolerating examinations, tests or procedures

Source: Adapted from Holz (1994), Kendall-Tackett (2003), and Roberts (1996)

opening this discussion as part of an effort to provide more comprehensive health care and that these questions are asked of all patients. For instance, when asking women about sexual assaults, the provider might say: "I talk to all of my patients about sexual assault because it is such a big problem in women's lives and it can hurt them in so many ways." Because many people are reluctant to assume the "abuse" label, the questions should ask whether they have experienced specific behaviors. For example, asking questions such as: "When you were a child did an adult ever touch you in a sexual manner?" tend to yield higher prevalence rates for sexual abuse than measures that label their experiences with emotionally laden terms such as "rape," "molestation," or "abuse" (Silvern *et al.*, 2000). Brochures about child abuse and domestic violence in the waiting room can also help patients feel comfortable discussing abuse with their provider (McCauley *et al.*, 1998). Conversely, not asking may inadvertently convey the message that an abuse history does not matter, or that abuse has no long-term effects and thus is not relevant to the patient's health (Holz, 1994).

Given that the co-occurrence of other types of maltreatment is common (Briere, 1992), a thorough trauma assessment should include questions regarding sexual, physical, psychological abuse, and neglect. If a positive history is obtained, the provider can then inquire about symptoms of depression, suicidality, self-mutilation, or posttraumatic stress disorder. Care should be taken not to ask pointed or invasive questions, and patients should be told to share only as much as they are comfortable with discussing at that moment. It should also be recognized that professional responses to disclosures can have a significant impact on the well-being of abuse victims. Unsupportive responses, such as those where professionals minimize, blame, or disbelieve victims' allegations of abuse appeared to exacerbate the negative effects. Such responses have been shown to hinder recovery in rape victims (Campbell *et al.*, 2001; Ullman, 1996) and are related to greater PTSD symptom severity (Ullman and Filipas, 2001). Supportive reactions, on the other hand, such as those where professionals acknowledge and validate victims' experiences, may help to mitigate the negative effects of abuse. A supportive response recommended by Draucker and Spradlin (2001, p. 45) is, "I can imagine it was hard for you to share that experience with me. I respect your courage for being able to do so."

Some abuse survivors will initially deny a victimization history. Barriers to disclosure include denial, shame, embarrassment, and fear of the reaction of others (McCauley *et al.*, 1998). However, even if patients choose not to disclose abuse they have experienced, the act of asking helps to "plant the seed," indicating that the health care provider takes the subject seriously (Holz, 1994). A study of pregnant women found that some did not reveal partner violence when initially screened, but disclosed after they had a developed a more trusting relationship with the health care provider (Lutz, 2005).

When asking about victimization, it is important to listen closely to what the patient has to say and recognize that many abuse victims will "test the waters" by revealing only a small portion of what has happened to them. If met with a supportive response, an abuse survivor may reveal more about what happened and how it has affected him or her. Because of the widespread and hidden nature of victimization, Tudiver *et al.* (2000) recommend that all medical personal adopt an approach of "universal precautions," which consider a possible history of prior abuse.

Evidence suggests that most women respond positively to being asked about victimization experiences by their provider. A group of researchers studied how young women responded to being asked about a sexual victimization history by their physician during routine care (Diaz *et al.*, 2004). In the great majority of the women (141 out of 146 patients), the physician was unaware of a history of sexual victimization. Of these 141 patients, 32 (23 percent) cases were identified. Almost all (93 percent) of these young women accepted referrals for on-site psychotherapy, and 81 percent kept their initial appointments. Diaz and colleagues concluded that many patients are willing to talk to health care providers about victimization and may be receptive to treatment of unresolved issues emanating from the abuse.

Schachter *et al.* (2004) asked 27 female childhood sexual abuse survivors about their experiences with health professionals and explored how practitioners could be more sensitive to their needs as survivors. The most predominant theme that emerged was the need to feel safe when interacting with health professionals. Survivors also wanted providers to share control and information with them. One of the most important ways providers can help an abuse survivor to feel more comfortable during office visits and procedures is to listen to what he or she wants (Kitzinger, 1992). In addition, because many survivors become anxious when faced with uncertainty, care should be taken to tell the patient what to expect during the visit. Retraumatization can be avoided by explaining upcoming procedures, encouraging patients to ask questions, and by giving survivors as much control as possible over what happens to them. If the patient is still anxious, the need for premedication or the presence of supportive others can be discussed (Roberts, 1996).

Because it is not always possible to take a victimization history prior to providing care, Tudiver *et al.* (2000) have recommended that all medical personnel adopt a policy of "universal precautions." When using this approach, providers would keep in mind the possibility of a background of victimization and routinely ask questions such as: "Do you have any special concerns about this procedure?" or "Is there anything that would make this examination more comfortable for you?" The provider should also check with patients during examinations or procedures to ask how they are doing. If the patient appears to be having a flashback or dissociative episode, it can be helpful to ask the patient to open his or her eyes and to focus on the "here and now." Chrestman and colleagues (1996) recommend drawing the patient's attention to the present surroundings by asking a question such as, "Will you tell me what you see on this wall?" If the patient revealed abuse during history-taking or experienced distress during the examination, it is important to check back on the survivor at the end of an appointment and ask how he or she is doing. Draucker and Spradlin (2001, p. 45), recommend saying: "For some women (men), sharing an abuse experience for the first time can result in some very strong (confusing, distressing) feelings. How are you feeling now? Are you feeling unsafe in any way?" If the patient appears to be having a difficult time, they should be provided with a referral to local resources such as a sexual assault center or community mental health facility.

CONCLUSION

Millions of people in our society are the victims of interpersonal violence at some point in their lives. Since primary care practitioners are often the first contact abuse victims have, they are in the best position to help victims of interpersonal violence. However, because providers rarely ask about abuse and survivors rarely volunteer this information, wounds from abuse typically remain concealed. Consequences of victimization include acute injuries and stress as well as long-term physical and mental health problems. An abuse history can also influence aspects of the health care encounter at every stage of the process. Abused patients may be estranged from their bodies and have difficulty interpreting symptoms. They may also respond with marked anxiety to procedures, examinations, or tests that contain reminders of the abuse. The main triggers involve touch, procedures involving previously traumatized parts of the body, feelings of vulnerability or exposure, feelings of uncertainty or a lack of control, and procedures that contain sensory elements reminiscent of the abuse. The abuse survivor may respond to such situations by dissociating, resulting in poor memory of the visit. A history of victimization can also lead to avoidance behaviors and influence the willingness of patients to comply with the recommendations of their health care provider.

By taking a victimization history and by being sensitive to how such history may be affecting their patients, providers can build trust and help alleviate some of the suffering associated with interpersonal violence. Much of retraumatization that abuse survivors experience in health care settings can be avoided by taking the time to explain upcoming procedures, by encouraging patients to ask questions, and by giving patients as much control as possible over what happens to them. To this end, medical personnel and support staff should be trained in the after-effects of interpersonal violence, and encouraged to exercise "universal precautions" that consider a possible history of prior victimization in all patients. Through adopting this approach, we can best heed Kitzinger's (1992) call for providers to try to ensure that the care they offer "*counteracts* rather than *reenacts*" the violence and violation that many patients have experienced in their lives (p. 220, emphasis in original).

REFERENCES

Aaron, L.A., and Buchwald, D. (2001). Fibromyalgia and other unexplained clinical conditions. *Current Rheumatology Reports, 3*, 116–122.

American Medical Association (1995). *Diagnostic and treatment guidelines on mental health effects of family violence*. Chicago, IL: Author.

American Psychiatric Association (1994). *Diagnostic and statistical manual for mental disorders* (4th edn). Washington, DC: Author.

Anda, R., Felitti, V., Bremner, J., Walker, J., Whitfield, C., Perry, B., *et al.* (2006). The enduring effects of abuse and related adverse experiences in childhood. *European Archives of Psychiatry and Clinical Neuroscience, 256*(3), 174–186.

Anonymous (2004). Dental phobia in survivors of sexual, emotional, or physical abuse. Downloaded on February 21, 2006 from http://www.dentalfearcentral.org/abuse_survivors.html.

Ballon, B.C., Courbasson, C.M., and Smith, P.D. (2001). Physical and sexual abuse issues among youths with substance use problems. *Canadian Journal of Psychiatry, 46,* 617–621.

Batten, S.V., Aslan, M., Maciejewski, P.K., and Mazure, C.M. (2004). Childhood maltreatment as a risk factor for adult cardiovascular disease and depression. *Journal of Clinical Psychiatry, 65,* 249–254.

Bergman, B., and Brismar, B. (1991). A 5-year follow-up study of 117 battered women. *American Journal of Public Health, 81,* 1486–1489.

Bohn, D.K., and Holz, K.A. (1996). Sequelae of abuse. Health effects of childhood sexual abuse, domestic battering, and rape. *Journal of Nurse Midwifery, 41,* 442–456.

Boisset-Pioro, M.H., Esdaile, J.M., and Fitzcharles, M.A. (1995). Sexual and physical abuse in women with fibromyalgia syndrome. *Arthritis and Rheumatism, 38,* 235–241.

Briere, J. (1992). *Child abuse trauma: Theory and treatment of the lasting effects.* Newbury Park, CA: Sage.

Briere, J., and Elliott, D.M. (2003). Prevalence and psychological sequelae of self-reported childhood physical and sexual abuse in a general population sample of men and women. *Child Abuse and Neglect, 27,* 1205–1222.

Briere, J., and Runtz, M. (1988). Symptomatology associated with childhood sexual victimization in a nonclinical adult sample. *Child Abuse and Neglect, 12,* 51–59.

Campbell, R., Ahrens, C.E., Sefl, T., Wasco, S.M., and Barnes, H.E. (2001). Social reactions to rape victims: Healing and hurtful effects on psychological and physical health outcomes. *Violence and Victims, 16,* 287–302.

Carlson, B.E., McNutt, L.A., and Choi, D.Y. (2003). Childhood and adult abuse among women in primary health care: Effects on mental health. *Journal of Interpersonal Violence, 18,* 924–941.

Centers for Disease Control (2003). Assessing health risk behaviors among young people: *Youth Risk Behavior Surveillance System*. Atlanta, GA: Author (online). Downloaded on February 21, 2006 from http://www.cdc.gov/nccdphp/aag/aag_yrbss.htm.

Chrestman, K.R., Prins, A., and Koss, M.P. (1996). Enhancement of primary care treatment for women trauma survivors. *National Center for PTSD Clinical Quarterly, 6*(4), 83–86. Downloaded on July 27, 2006 from http://www.ncptsd.va.gov/publications/cq/v6/n4/chrestma.html.

Courtois, C.A. (1988). *Healing the incest wound*. New York: W.W. Norton.

Courtois, C.A., and Riley, C. (1992). Pregnancy and childbirth as triggers for abuse memories: Implications for care. *Birth, 19*, 222–223.

Crofford, L. (1996). The hypothalamic-pituitary-adrenal axis in the fibromyalgia syndrome. *Journal of Musculoskeletal Pain, 4*, 181–200.

Dallam, S.J. (1997). The identification and management of self-mutilating patients in primary care. *The Nurse Practitioner, 22*, 151–165.

Dallam, S.J. (2001). The long-term medical consequences of childhood trauma. In K. Franey, R. Geffner, and R. Falconer (eds), *The cost of child maltreatment: Who pays? We all do* (pp. 1–14). San Diego, CA: Family Violence and Sexual Assault Institute.

Dallam, S.J. (2005). Health issues associated with violence against women. In K. Kendall-Tackett (ed.). *The handbook of women, stress, and trauma* (pp. 159–180). New York: Brunner-Routledge.

De Bellis, M.D. (2002). Developmental traumatology: A contributory mechanism for alcohol and substance use disorders. *Psychoneuroendocrinology. 27*, 155–170.

Diaz, A., Simatov, E., and Rickert, V.I. (2000). The independent and combined effects of physical and sexual abuse on health. Results of a national survey. *Journal of Pediatric and Adolescent Gynecology, 13*, 89.

Diaz, A., Edwards, S., Neal, W.P., Ludmer, P., Sondike, S.B., Kessler, C., *et al.* (2004). Obtaining a history of sexual victimization from adolescent females seeking routine health care. *Mount Sinai Journal of Medicine, 71*, 170–173.

Domino, J.V., and Haber, J.D. (1987). Prior physical and sexual abuse in women with chronic headache: Clinical correlates. *Headache, 27*, 310–314.

Draucker, C.B., and Spradlin, D. (2001). Women sexually abused as children: Implications for orthopaedic nursing care. *Orthopedic Nursing, 20*(6), 41–48.

Drossman, D.A., Leserman, J., Nachman, G., Li, Z.M., Gluck, H., Toomey, T.C., *et al.* (1990). Sexual and physical abuse in women with functional or organic gastrointestinal disorders. *Annals of Internal Medicine, 113*, 828–833.

Dube, S.R., Felitti, V.J., Dong, M., Chapman, D.P., Giles, W.H., and Anda, R.F. (2003). Childhood abuse, neglect, and household dysfunction and the risk of illicit drug use: The adverse childhood experiences study. *Pediatrics, 111*, 564–572.

Family Violence Prevention Fund (2004). *National consensus guidelines on identifying and responding to domestic violence victimization in health care settings*. San Francisco, CA: Author.

Farley, M., and Patsalides, B.M. (2001). Physical symptoms, posttraumatic stress disorder, and healthcare utilization of women with and without childhood physical and sexual abuse. *Psychological Reports, 89*, 595–606.

Felitti, V.J. (1991). Long-term medical consequences of incest, rape, and molestation. *Southern Medical Journal, 84*, 328–331.

Felitti, V.J. (2002). The relationship between adverse childhood experiences and adult health: Turning gold into lead. *The Permanente Journal, 6*(1), 44–47.

Felitti, V.J., Anda, R.F., Nordenberg, D., Williamson, D.F., Spitz, A.M., Edwards, V., Koss, M.P., and Marks, J.S. (1998). Relationship of childhood abuse and household dysfunction to many of the leading causes of death in adults. The Adverse Childhood Experiences (ACE) Study. *American Journal of Preventive Medicine, 14*, 245–258.

Fergusson, D.M., Horwood, L.J., and Lynskey, M.T. (1997). Childhood sexual abuse, adolescent sexual behaviors and sexual revictimization. *Child Abuse and Neglect, 21*, 789–803.

Florida Council Against Sexual Violence (2002). *How to screen your patients for sexual assault: A guide for health care professionals*. Tallahassee, FL: Author.

Ford, J.D., Ruzek, J.I., and Niles, B.L. (1996). Identifying and treating VA medical care patients with undetected sequelae of psychological trauma and post-traumatic stress disorder. *National Center for PTSD Clinical Quarterly, 6*(4), 77–82.

Girdler, S.S., Pedersen, C.A., Straneva, P.A., Leserman, J., Stanwyck. C.L., Benjamin, S., and Light, K.C. (1998). Dysregulation of cardiovascular and neuroendocrine responses to stress in premenstrual dysphoric disorder. *Psychiatry Research, 81*, 163–178.

Girdler, S.S., Sherwood, A., Hinderliter, A.L., Leserman, J., Costello, N.L., Straneva, P.A., *et al.* (2003). Biological correlates of abuse in women with premenstrual dysphoric disorder and healthy controls. *Psychosomatic Medicine, 65*, 849–856.

Golding, J.M., Cooper, M.L., and George, L.K. (1997). Sexual assault history and health perceptions: Seven general population studies. *Health Psychology, 16*, 417–425.

Gracely, R.H., Petzke, F., Wolf, J.M., and Clauw, D.J. (2002). Functional magnetic resonance imaging evidence of augmented pain processing in fibromyalgia. *Arthritis and Rheumatism, 46*(5), 1333–1343.

Green, B.L., Krupnick, J.L., Rowland, J.H., Epstein, S.A., Stockton, P., Spertus, I., and Stern, N. (2000). Trauma history as a predictor of psychologic symptoms in women with breast cancer. *Journal of Clinical Oncology, 18*, 1084–1093.

Gutman, D.A., and Nemeroff, C.B. (2003). Persistent central nervous system effects of an adverse early environment: Clinical and preclinical studies. *Physiology and Behavior, 79*, 471–478.

Haas, B., and Popp, F. (2006). Why do people injure themselves? *Psychopathology, 39*, 10–18.

Hall, M.A., Zheng, B., Dugan, E., Camacho, F., Kidd, K.E., Mishra, A., *et al.* (2002). Measuring patients' trust in their primary care providers. *Medical Care Research and Review, 59*, 293–318.

Harrison, P.A., Hoffmann, N.G., and Edwall, G.E. (1989). Differential drug use patterns among sexually abused adolescent girls in treatment for chemical dependency. *International Journal of Addictions, 24*, 499–514.

Harrop-Griffiths, J., Katon, W., Walker, E., Holm, L., Russo, J., and Hickok, L. (1988). The association between chronic pelvic pain, psychiatric diagnoses, and childhood sexual abuse. *Obstetrics and Gynecology, 71*, 589–594.

Heim, C., Ehlert, U., Hanker, J.P., and Hellhammer, D.H. (1998). Abuse-related posttraumatic stress disorder and alterations of the hypothalamic-pituitary-adrenal axis in women with chronic pelvic pain. *Psychosomatic Medicine, 60*, 309–318.

Holz, K.A. (1994). A practical approach to clients who are survivors of childhood sexual abuse. *Journal of Nurse Midwifery, 39*, 13–18.

Horowitz, M.J. (1986). *Stress response syndromes* (2nd edn). New York: Jason Aronson.

Imbierowicz, K., and Egle, U.T. (2003). Childhood adversities in patients with fibromyalgia and somatoform pain disorder. *European Journal of Pain, 7*, 113–119.

Kendall-Tackett, K. (2003). *Treating the lifetime health effects of childhood victimization*. Kingston, NJ: Civic Research Institute.

Kendler, K.S., Bulik, C.M., Silberg, J., Hettema, J.M., Myers, J., and Prescott, C.A. (2000). Childhood sexual abuse and adult psychiatric and substance use disorders in women: An epidemiological and cotwin control analysis. *Archives of General Psychiatry, 57*, 953–959.

Kiecolt-Glaser, J.K., Preacher, K.J., MacCallum, R.C., Atkinson, C., Malarkey, W.B., and Glaser, R. (2003). Chronic stress and age-related increases in the proinflammatory cytokine IL-6. *Proceedings of the National Academy of Sciences, USA, 100*, 9090–9095.

Kilpatrick, D.G., Acierno, R., Resnick, H.S., Saunders, B.E., and Best, C.L. (1997). A 2-year longitudinal analysis of the relationships between violent assault and substance use in women. *Journal of Consulting and Clinical Psychology, 65*, 834–847.

Kitzinger, J. (1992). Counteracting, not reenacting, the violation of women's bodies: The challenge for perinatal caregivers. *Birth, 198*, 219–221.

Koss, M.P., Woodruff, W.J., and Koss, P.G. (1990). Relation of criminal victimization to health perceptions among women medical patients. *Journal of Consulting and Clinical Psychology, 58*, 147–152.

Lechner, M.E., Vogel, M.E., Garcia-Shelton, L.M., Leichter, J.L., and Steibel, K.R. (1993). Self-reported medical problems of adult female survivors of childhood sexual abuse. *Journal of Family Practice, 36*, 633–638.

Leserman, J., Li, Z., Hu, Y.J., and Drossman, D.A. (1998). How multiple types of stressors impact on health. *Psychosomatic Medicine, 60*, 175–181.

Linton, S.J. (1997). A population-based study of the relationship between sexual abuse and back pain: Establishing a link. *Pain, 73*, 47–53.

Lutz, K.F. (2005). Abuse experiences, perceptions, and associated decisions during the childbearing cycle. *Western Journal of Nursing Research, 27*, 802–824.

Mazza, D., Dennerstein, L., and Ryan, V. (1996). Physical, sexual and emotional violence against women: A general practice–based prevalence study. *Medical Journal of Australia, 164*, 14–17.

McCauley, J., Yurk, R., Jenckes, M., and Ford, D. (1998). Inside "Pandora's box": Abused women's experiences with clinicians and health services. *Archives of Internal Medicine, 13*, 549–555.

McNutt, L.A., van Ryn, M., Clark, C., and Fraiser, I. (2000). Partner violence and medical encounters: African-American women's perspectives. *American Journal of Preventive Medicine, 19*, 264–269.

Milla, P.J. (2001). Irritable bowel syndrome in childhood. *Gastroenterology, 120*, 287–290.

Moeller, T.P., Bachmann, G.A., and Moeller, J.R. (1993). The combined effects of physical, sexual, and emotional abuse during childhood: Long-term health consequences for women. *Child Abuse and Neglect, 17*, 623–640.

Molnar, B.E., Buka, S.L., and Kessler, R.C. (2001). Child sexual abuse and subsequent psychopathology: Results from the National Comorbidity Survey. *American Journal of Public Health, 91*, 753–760.

Morse, D.S., Suchman, A.L., and Frankel, R.M. (1997). The meaning of symptoms in 10 women with somatization disorder and a history of childhood abuse. *Archives of Family Medicine, 6*, 468–476.

Penza, K.M., Heim, C., and Nemeroff, C.B. (2003). Neurobiological effects of childhood abuse: Implications for the pathophysiology of depression and anxiety. *Archives of Women's Mental Health, 6*, 15–22.

Perry, B.D. (2000). Trauma and terror in childhood: The neuropsychiatric impact of childhood trauma. In I. Schulz, S. Carella, and D.O. Brady (eds), *Handbook of psychological injuries: Evaluation, treatment and compensable damages.* Washington, DC: American Bar Association Publishing.

Perry, B.D., and Azad, I. (1999). Post-traumatic stress disorders in children and adolescents. *Current Opinion in Pediatrics. 11*, 121–132.

Perry, B.D., Pollard, R., Blakely, T., Baker, W., and Vigilante, D. (1995). Childhood trauma, the neurobiology of adaptation and "use-dependent" development of the brain: How "states" become "traits." *Infant Mental Health Journal, 16*, 271–291.

Plichta, S.B. (1992). The effects of woman abuse on health care utilization and health status: A literature review. *Women's Health Issues, 2*, 154–163.

Plichta, S.B., and Falik, M. (2001). Prevalence of violence and its implications for women's health. *Women's Health Issues. 11*, 244–258.

Raj, A., Silverman, J.G., and Amaro, H. (2000). The relationship between sexual abuse and sexual risk among high school students: Findings from the 1997 Massachusetts Youth Risk Behavior Survey. *Maternal and Child Health Journal, 4*, 125–134.

Reiter, R.C., Shakerin, L.R., Gambone, J.C., and Milburn, A.K. (1991). Correlation between sexual abuse and somatization in women with somatic and nonsomatic chronic pelvic pain. *American Journal of Obstetrics and Gynecology, 165*, 104–109.

Roberts, S.J. (1996). The sequelae of childhood sexual abuse: A primary care focus for adult female survivors. *Nurse Practitioner, 21*(12), 42–52.

Romans, S., Belaise, C., Martin, J., Morris, E., and Raffi, A. (2002). Childhood abuse and later medical disorders in women. An epidemiological study. *Psychotherapy and Psychosomatics, 71*, 141–150.

Salmon, P., and Calderbank, S. (1996). The relationship of childhood physical and sexual abuse to adult illness behavior. *Journal of Psychosomatic Research, 40*, 329–336.

Schachter, C.L., Stalker, C., and Teram, E. (1999). Toward sensitive practice: Issues for physical therapists working with survivors of childhood sexual abuse. *Physical Therapy, 79*, 248–261.

Schachter, C.L., Radomsky, N.S., Stalker, C., and Teram, E. (2004). Women survivors of child sexual abuse: How can health professionals promote healing? *Canadian Family Physician, 50*, 405–412.

Seng, J.S., Sparbel, K.J., Low, L.K., and Killion, C. (2002). Abuse-related posttraumatic stress and desired maternity care practices: Women's perspectives. *Journal of Midwifery and Women's Health, 47*, 360–370.

Silvern, L., Waelde, L.C., Baughan, B.M., Karyl, J., and Kaersvang, L.L. (2000). Two formats for eliciting retrospective reports of child sexual and physical abuse: Effects on apparent prevalence and relationships to adjustment. *Child Maltreatment, 5*, 236–250.

Spiegel, D., and Cardena, E. (1991). Disintegrated experience: The dissociative disorders revisited. *Journal of Abnormal Psychology, 100*, 366–378.

Springs, F.E., and Friedrich, W.N. (1992). Health risk behaviors and medical sequelae of childhood sexual abuse. *Mayo Clinic Proceedings, 67*, 527–532.

Stalker, C.A., Russell, B.D., Teram, E., and Schachter, C.L. (2005). Providing dental care to survivors of childhood sexual abuse: Treatment considerations for the practitioner. *Journal of the American Dental Association, 136*, 1277–1281.

Stein, M.B., and Barrett-Connor, E. (2000). Sexual assault and physical health: Findings from a population-based study of older adults. *Psychosomatic Medicine, 62*, 838–843.

Swahnberg, K., Wijma, B., Wingren, G., Hilden, M., and Schei, B. (2004). Women's perceived experiences of abuse in the health care system: Their relationship to childhood abuse. *British Journal of Obstetrics and Gynecology. 111*, 1429–1436.

Tang, B., Jamieson, E., Boyle, M., Libby, A., Gafni, A., and Macmillan, H. (in press). The influence of child abuse on the pattern of expenditures in women's adult health service utilization in Ontario, Canada. *Social Science and Medicine*.

Teicher, M.H. (2002). Scars that won't heal: The neurobiology of child abuse. *Scientific American, 286*, 68–75.

Tudiver, S., McClure, L., Heinonen, T., Scurfield, C. and Kreklewetz, C. (2000). Women survivors of childhood sexual abuse: Knowledge and preparation of health care providers to meet client needs. Report of research for the Women's Health Bureau of Health Canada through the Prairie Women's Health Centre of Excellence. Downloaded on July 12, 2006 from http://www.cwhn.ca/resources/csa/abuse.pdf.

Ullman, S.E. (1996). Social reactions, coping strategies, and self-blame attributions in adjustment to sexual assault. *Psychology of Women Quarterly, 20*, 505–526.

Ullman, S.E., and Filipas, H.H. (2001). Predictors of PTSD symptom severity and social reactions in sexual assault victims. *Journal of Traumatic Stress, 14*, 393–413.

Walker, E.A., Torkelson, N., Katon, W.J., and Koss, M.P. (1993). The prevalence rate of sexual trauma in a primary care clinic. *Journal of the American Board of Family Practice, 6*, 465–471.

Walker, E.A., Gelfand, A., Katon, W.J., Koss, M.P., Von Korff, M., Bernstein, D., *et al.* (1999a). Adult health status of women with histories of childhood abuse and neglect. *American Journal of Medicine, 107*, 332–339.

Walker, E.A., Unutzer, J., Rutter, C., Gelfand, A., Saunders, K., VonKorff, M., *et al.* (1999b). Costs of health care use by women HMO members with a history of childhood abuse and neglect. *Archives of General Psychiatry, 56*, 609–613.

Whitehead, W.E., Palsson, O., and Jones, K.R. (2002). Systematic review of the comorbidity of irritable bowel syndrome with other disorders: What are the causes and implications? *Gastroenterology, 122*, 1140–1156.

Client-centered care

Integrating the perspectives of childhood sexual abuse survivors and clinicians

Carol A. Stalker, Candice L. Schachter,
Eli Teram, and Gerri C. Lasiuk

BETWEEN 1990 AND 1994, Candice Schachter, a physical therapist, worked as a volunteer in a community-based sexual assault center. She served as a lay co-facilitator with a professional social worker providing group support for women survivors of childhood sexual abuse (CSA). In this role, Candice listened to women talk about the difficulties they experienced when seeking health care. Some talked about being afraid to consult a health professional (HP) because they anticipated not being able to tolerate the examination and treatment processes. One woman talked about going to a practitioner on one occasion and having such a negative experience that she could not return. Candice recognized that physical therapists and other HPs, trained to focus on the health of the body rather than on mental health, had not been taught that CSA could have this kind of impact on survivors' abilities to access health care. The result was a series of collaborations, one of which is the subject of this chapter. In particular, we focus on qualitative research aimed at describing male and female CSA survivors' experiences with health professionals. Our aims were to listen to and learn from survivors about their experiences with HPs and to collaborate with both survivors and HPs to identify principles of "sensitive practice."

THE RELATIONSHIP BETWEEN CLIENT-CENTERED AND SENSITIVE PRACTICE

Patient- or client-centered care is a concept that has been embraced by many health care professions. Existing research links elements of patient-centered care with both increased patient satisfaction and improved patient outcomes (e.g., Little *et al.*, 2001; Safran *et al.*, 1998; Stewart, 1995; Stewart *et al.*, 2001). A patient/client-centered approach recognizes and responds compassionately to the vulnerability that all human beings experience when they are ill, in pain, or uncertain about their health and well-being (e.g., Powers *et al.*, 2000; Stewart *et al.*, 1995, 2003). For us, sensitive practice is behavior and attitudes that allow HPs to be with, and work with survivors in ways that are sensitive to their particular needs. The principles and guidelines of sensitive practice contribute to a client-centered approach by providing specific guidance on how HPs can work effectively and ethically with individuals who have a history of CSA.

DEFINITION AND PREVALENCE OF CSA AND RESEARCH LINKING CSA AND HEALTH PROBLEMS

In all countries where it has been studied, a notable percentage of the adult population has reported a history of CSA (Finkelhor, 1994a). Because of the criminal and stigmatizing nature of CSA it is not possible to know the prevalence of this experience in the general population with certainty. However, Finkelhor (1994b) concludes that CSA affects approximately 20 percent of women and 5 percent to 10 percent of men.

The Adverse Childhood Experiences (ACE) study found that ACEs were strongly associated with increased prevalence of the major causes of death and disability in the United States (Felitti *et al.*, 1998). Similarly, Walker and colleagues (1999a) found that abuse survivors had poorer perceptions of their overall health, greater physical and emotional functional disability, more physical health symptoms, and more health risk behaviors than those without such a history. Kendall-Tackett (2002) has argued that a complex combination of behavioural, emotional, social, and cognitive factors mediates the relationship between childhood abuse and later health problems.

CSA survivors have higher rates of chronic pelvic pain, gastrointestinal disorders, irritable bowel syndrome and recurrent headaches than comparison groups (e.g., Felitti, 1991; Harrop-Griffiths *et al.*, 1988; Lampe *et al.*, 2000; Reiter and Gambone, 1990; Walker *et al.*, 1988, 1993). In community samples, CSA survivors also have higher rates of chronic fatigue, asthma, and cardiovascular problems (Romans *et al.*, 2002), and were more likely to have poor perceptions of their general health, sustained a serious injury in adulthood, had a miscarriage or stillbirth, acquired a chronic mental health condition in adulthood, and recently used drugs (Thompson *et al.*, 2002).

Numerous studies have also found an association between a history of CSA and increased use of medical services (Arnow *et al.*, 1999; Hulme, 2000; Leserman *et al.*, 1998; Newman *et al.*, 2000; Sickel *et al.*, 2002; Walker *et al.*, 1999b). One of the limitations of much of this research is that it has focused primarily on women; few samples include males in spite of increasing awareness that sexual abuse occurs to significant numbers of boys and is as harmful to male children as it is to female children (Finkelhor, 1994b).

The available evidence, therefore, strongly suggests that the proportion of a health professional's clients with a history of CSA may be larger than the proportion one would see in the general population. The research linking CSA, health problems, and health care utilization as well as research exploring the body's neurobiological responses to traumatic stress (Yehuda, 2001) is relatively recent, and many HPs may not be aware of this information or its implications for their practice. The research we describe in this chapter was motivated by the desire to increase health professionals' ability to work effectively with their patients/clients who had been traumatized by CSA.

RESEARCH METHODOLOGY

Our intent in this research was not simply to document survivors' experiences with HPs, but to engage in a process by which survivors and HPs could both contribute to knowledge development and influence health care practices. The first study was implemented in three phases using grounded theory (Glaser and Strauss, 1967) and action research (Reason and Bradbury, 2001) methods, and we interviewed 27 women from Saskatchewan and Ontario who had received physical therapy or who had been referred for physical therapy. We asked the women to talk about their experiences, feelings, and concerns with respect to interactions with physical therapists and other "touch" practitioners such as chiropractors and massage therapists. To ensure that our theory reflected participants' reality, we sent a summary of our interpretation of the data to them and incorporated their responses regarding inaccuracies and other suggestions.

In the second phase, two separate "working groups," each composed of four women survivors and four physical therapists, met together once a month for approximately six months to transform the findings from the interviews into concrete suggestions and guidelines for sensitive practice. In phase three, we asked all participants from phases one and two to provide written feedback on the first draft. The first edition of the *Handbook on sensitive practice for health professionals: Lessons from women survivors of childhood sexual abuse*, was published by Health Canada in 2001 (Schachter *et al.*, 2001).

In the process of conducting this first study, it became clear that many of the suggestions and recommendations for sensitive practice were applicable to all HPs, not only to physical therapists. The recognition that the principles had relevance for all HPs led to a decision to extend the study to male survivors and a broader range of HPs.

Our second study was designed to address questions and gaps that emerged from the first study. We interviewed 49 male survivors individually and talked with nine men in a group setting. We also interviewed 19 women survivors and specifically asked about their experiences with all HPs including physicians, nurses, nurse practitioners, dentists, chiropractors, massage therapists, and so on (other than mental health professionals).

As in the first study, transcripts were sent to participants inviting corrections and feedback, and a similar process to the first study was followed. Working groups of male survivors and physicians, male survivors and nurses/nurse practitioners, female survivors and physicians and female survivors and nurses were facilitated. A second edition of the *Handbook* (Schachter *et al.*, in press), which is more inclusive than the first, is currently in press and will be available on the Public Health Agency of Canada's National Clearinghouse on Family Violence website in Fall 2008. See http://www.phac-aspc.gc.ca/ncfv-cnivf.familyviolence/ index.html. We would like to emphasize the parallel that exists between the collaborative nature of our research process and the client-centered care that the findings support. Many survivors told us about the importance for them of sharing power in their interactions with HPs. They emphasized their sensitivity to behaviors that suggest a lack of respect, devaluing, or dismissal of their concerns and their need to have a sense of control in their interactions with HPs. Throughout our research, we have been committed to a process that recognizes and incorporates the expertise of both survivors and HPs.

HOW CSA CAN AFFECT SURVIVORS AND THE HEALTH CARE ENCOUNTER

Survivors of CSA are a heterogeneous group, and while research findings associate CSA with a wide range of psychological, interpersonal, and physical health problems in adulthood, not all survivors live with symptoms of ill health or other forms of distress (Fergusson and Mullen, 1999). The intrusiveness and duration of the abuse, the degree of coercion or violence, the relationship with the perpetrator, the extent of family support and exposure to other forms of abuse have all been shown to affect the long-term sequelae of abuse (Fergusson and Mullen, 1999). Furthermore, the degree to which encounters with HPs are affected by an individual's history of abuse will depend on where the individual is in the recovery process.

That said, the participants in our studies talked about a great number of experiences that are affected by their histories of abuse; in fact, they reported that many of the difficulties described in the literature as being associated with past abuse are often triggered in health care encounters. Below, we briefly summarize the difficulties that survivors in our studies experienced in their encounters with health professionals and attributed to their histories of CSA. For more information about how a history of CSA can affect survivors, please refer to the *Handbook* (Schachter *et al.*, in press).

FEAR, ANXIETY, LACK OF TRUST, AND DISSOCIATIVE EPISODES

Many of the survivors described intense feelings of fear, anxiety, and lack of trust as they anticipated their meetings with HPs. These feelings often centered around having to undress, a sense of vulnerability at having their bodies exposed under skimpy gowns, and being touched. Some survivors described dissociative episodes or flashbacks and not always knowing what might trigger such reactions. Many, however, knew that being required to assume a certain body position or having a pelvic, genital, or rectal examination were likely to trigger a negative experience. Another common theme was a generalized distrust of authority figures, often articulated as fear that HPs (as powerful others) would be disrespectful, controlling, or even abusive. For a number of survivors, seeing an HP who is the same gender as their abuser(s) was especially problematic. Still other survivors told us about their complete inability to tolerate visits with HPs and described their strategies of avoidance (for example, frequently making and cancelling appointments or completely refusing to seek care despite acknowledged health problems).

DIFFICULTY ASSERTING THEMSELVES, AMBIVALENCE ABOUT THE BODY, FEELING UNDESERVING

The survivors in our studies described difficulty asserting themselves and participating in examinations or treatment. As one man said,

> "You see one of the other things with people who have been abused . . . is they're scared of authority figures, number one, and they can't say no, number two . . . so [HPs] really have to listen between the lines."

Many survivors expressed ambivalence towards their bodies, feelings of hate, guilt, and shame about their bodies, and/or their struggles to take care of their bodies. This was often associated with a belief that they were undeserving of being treated well and of difficulty following recommendations that they knew would benefit their health.

PAIN

For many survivors, pain was a complicated combination of acute and chronic conditions (some resulting from past abuse) and somatization. According to another male survivor,

> "some men say that they have experiences of pain that they find hard to sort out [in terms of the cause] between things they've experienced in the past and things that are going on now."

Some participants referred to the mind/body connection involving the combination of emotional pain from past abuse, the physical pain that may have resulted from past abuse, and current health issues.

A female survivor said,

> "I think there is a mind/body connection. I think [going to a HP] for a physical ailment, there's more than just the physical hurt, unless of course you break a bone or you twist your ankle. I mean there's the obvious what you can see and there's the other pain, physical pain versus mental pain, emotional pain."

The fear and anxiety associated with encounters with a HP visit often fueled the pain, and the pain sometimes triggered memories of abuse.

PRINCIPLES OF SENSITIVE PRACTICE

SENSITIVE PRACTICE AS "UNIVERSAL PRECAUTIONS"
A CSA history can affect interactions with HPs in multiple ways. Much of the time, HPs are not aware that they are working with a survivor of CSA. For this reason, we advocate that HPs follow the principles of sensitive practice with all clients. The fundamental principles of professionalism, as articulated by the Physician Charter (Project of the ABIM Foundation, ACP-ASIM Foundation, and European Federation of Internal Medicine, 2002) – namely, primacy of patient welfare, patient autonomy, and social justice – can only be upheld by the use of sensitive practice in a conscious and deliberate way. Indeed, our findings, and those of other researchers (Monahan and Forgash, 2000; Schachter *et al.*, 1999, 2004; Seng *et al.*, 2002; Stalker, 1999, 2005; Teram *et al.*, 2006) suggest that losing sight of sensitive practice can be retraumatizing and harmful to the health and well-being of many survivors. One man said,

> "This may be a person who's gone through something very traumatic . . . [who needs] . . . some real safe technique . . . [like] asking permission to proceed. Because otherwise you're going to have a certain segment of patients that are going to walk away feeling as though they've been abused all over again, quietly abused, just walking away and seeking another health care practitioner, just going through the cycle, again and again and again and maybe not understanding why, maybe not knowing how to say it, how to voice that, just keep going through that whole cycle over and over again.. There's a huge populous out there that just needs that extra gentle care. It's because of that, maybe the whole populous needs to be treated the same way."

SENSE OF SAFETY: THE OVERARCHING CONSIDERATION
Participants in both of our studies emphasized that safety is the
crucial element in all client–clinician interactions. We have
conceptualized safety as a protective umbrella held open by the
nine principles of sensitive practice, which serve as the "spokes"
of the umbrella. The nine principles of sensitive practice are:
respect, rapport, taking time, sharing information, sharing control,
respecting boundaries, fostering mutual learning, understanding
that healing is not a linear process, and demonstrating awareness
and knowledge about trauma and interpersonal violence.
Figure 7.1 is a visual representation of the safety umbrella.

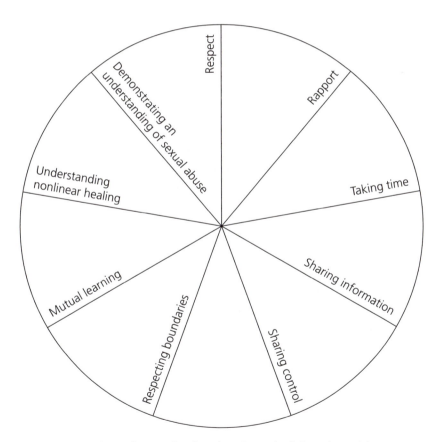

FIGURE 7.1 The safety umbrella. The nine principles of sensitive
practice keep the umbrella of safety open, maximizing the benefit
survivors of CSA receive from the health care encounter.

RESPECT

Remembering that abuse is fundamentally disrespectful, it is not surprising that many survivors talked about being very sensitive to any hint of disrespect. One man said,

"[Feeling respected] to the person who has been abused, it certainly means a great deal. And when you are treated in a demeaning fashion . . . I would think even [for] an ordinary person it's harmful to your sense of self."

A woman participant said,

"It's critical that they [HPs] understand that we can be retraumatized as a result of how we are treated by them. . . . Not that they're meaning to go there but by not treating us respectfully, giving us what we need to feel safe and being allowed to be seen as co-partnering and not as having no power at all, that it's possible for us to be retraumatized."

RAPPORT

Even though establishing and maintaining rapport is important in every therapeutic relationship, for the CSA survivor it is essential to feelings of safety. Developing rapport begins at the first moment of clinician–client interaction and requires ongoing attention. Participants told how the combination of respect and rapport helped them to feel that the HP cared about them as a human being. One man said,

"[At times when I have seen a HP] I've felt . . . like an object. Which brings back memories because a lot of the sexual abuse made me feel like an object rather than like a human being. So, when the [exam] is done just like [I'm] an object then it brings back flashbacks.

TAKING TIME

Participants were keenly aware of the time pressures on health providers; they said they would welcome a discussion about how to best use the time together. They told us that it is a powerful experience when an HP takes the time to establish a positive connection and to really listen to what they have to say. A man said,

> "It's the [HPs] that . . . stop and give you a moment. And that's one of the biggest healing things right there, that moment."

Participants spoke of feeling objectified when their encounters with HPs were rushed; this could exacerbate feelings of distrust and anxiety. For some, it could trigger a dissociative episode or a flashback. Participants strongly urged clinicians to openly discuss and negotiate time issues with them.

SHARING INFORMATION

Participants overwhelmingly stressed the importance of HPs sharing information with them in ways that they could understand. They want to be informed about what an examination involves, why it is being done, the implications of the findings, and their treatment options. As one woman explained,

> "For me, it's fear, anxiety and fear of not knowing what will happen next. I think, as a survivor, one tends to have more anxiety over some of these things. People coming around and touching you or not explaining there is uncertainty as to what's going to happen next type thing and why are they not conferring with me and why are they not asking, 'Is this okay?' "

Another woman said,

> "He doesn't overdo it, but he explains everything he does, so that I have a very clear sense of where he's going and what he's doing next. And this has been extremely helpful."

A male survivor reiterated that,

> "surprises are the worst thing. They may be doing perfectly legitimate things but if it catches me off guard . . . that's anxiety causing."

Participants also emphasized that the sharing of information needs to be a reciprocal process with the HP sharing information with the client and seeking information from the survivor about her or his body, reactions to treatment and her or his ongoing comfort level. As one man framed it,

> "Before [starting] . . . they should lay the ground [rules]. 'How can I make you more comfortable here? . . . If there's something I'm doing, the way I'm touching you . . . makes you feel uncomfortable, let me know . . . Anything at all that would make you feel uncomfortable in this room, let me know.' That would be great. For myself, that would really open the door for me to say, 'Hey, maybe this is a safe place . . . maybe I'll stick with this physiotherapist and make myself feel better.' "

SHARING CONTROL

As children, survivors of abuse had little control over their bodies (i.e., others acted on their bodies without their consent). Participants told us how important it was for them to avoid feeling helpless or out of control. They stressed that their sense of safety and their ability to tolerate interactions with the HP are bolstered when control is shared. They need clinicians to provide information, to solicit information and feedback, and to negotiate a mutually acceptable course of action. One woman said,

> "The [physical therapist] would sort of tell me [what she wanted to do] and sort of show on herself, and then she'd ask am I comfortable with this? . . . [And before each step] she'd ask me again . . . so she gave me an opportunity that, if I were to change my mind and feel uncomfortable, all of a sudden, for whatever reason, she would know, and I'd be able to say something. So I felt like I was in control, and I did have the say of what was going on"[1] (p. 254).

Another woman told us,

> "It's the approach for me. That immediate taking over,

taking over for me without consulting me or giving me a choice . . . [F]or me that's the first thing that raises my anxiety level a little bit . . . for instance, if you lay on a table, [the HP could say] 'Are you okay to lay sideways or are you okay to lay on your back?' Instead of telling me 'You lay on your back'."

RESPECTING BOUNDARIES

The word "boundaries" refers to the outer limit of personal space (physical, psychological, emotional, and spiritual) under our control. Boundary violations occur not only when HPs disregard the client's boundaries but also when the clinician places his or her needs above those of the client (such as when an HP, rushed for time, begins an exam without obtaining consent). Participants in our studies emphasized that their sense of safety was highly affected by the clinician's awareness of and respect for their personal space. For this reason, the principles of sensitive practice incorporate both respect in general and respect of boundaries in particular. One survivor participant told us,

> "As a survivor, I need to know that that person is not going to invade my space. Or do harm to me. Not necessarily physically, but emotionally"[2] (p. 14).

In contrast, when boundaries are disregarded, health care interventions can be retraumatizing. A male survivor said,

> "He just began working, without saying what he was doing or what was going on, so I just felt . . . well, it felt like abuse all over again."

FOSTERING A MUTUAL LEARNING PROCESS

It is important to recognize that both the survivor and the HP learn as they work together. Survivors told us about gaining greater understanding of how their abuse experiences affected them and about learning new ways to take care of themselves and respond in health care settings. For example, some recognized that they had been conditioned to accept and never question the directions of authority figures. These survivors needed repeated invitations and encouragement to participate in their health care and to learn that it was safe to express their own feelings and wishes. One woman said,

> "That assertiveness of [saying] 'no' takes a long time to get . . . it was somebody else giving me permission that allowed me to say 'no' until I could learn to give myself permission [to do so]"[1] (p. 254).

Learning is ongoing for the HP as well. Because no set of responses will be "correct" for every survivor, mistakes and misunderstandings are bound to occur. When this happens it is best for the clinician to acknowledge the problem and discuss it with the client.

UNDERSTANDING THAT HEALING IS NOT A LINEAR PROCESS

Neither living with the effects nor healing from childhood sexual abuse are linear processes. As a result, survivors' abilities to tolerate and participate in treatment can vary widely over time. These variations may occur day to day or over weeks or months. In recognition of this, the clinician must repeatedly "check in" with the client and endeavor to adjust their approach accordingly. One woman said,

> "Parts of my body at different times might be untouchable. It's gonna change, depending on what I'm dealing with. So, you're not going to be able to make a list and count on that every time kinda thing: it's gonna be a check-in every session"[1] (p. 255).

The cost of ignoring this variability can run high – clinicians may feel frustrated and label the survivor as "difficult," while the survivor's sense of safety may be shaken to the point that she or he cannot continue working with the HP. One woman said,

> "I'm learning that if I don't have a sense of control . . . I will walk away from [the situation]"[1] (p. 255).

**DEMONSTRATING AWARENESS AND KNOWLEDGE ABOUT
INTERPERSONAL VIOLENCE AND TRAUMA**

Many survivors told us that they look for indicators of a clinician's awareness of issues related to interpersonal violence and trauma. Demonstrating this awareness can take a variety of forms. For example, posters and pamphlets from local organizations that work with individuals who have experienced violence are a cue that an HP has such an awareness of the prevalence and sequelae of interpersonal violence. One woman said,

> **"I'm way more interested in . . . how much awareness
> [the HP has] around trauma. So, that holds a lot of
> weight with me"**[2] (p. 16).

A male participant stressed that male survivors need messages that are specifically geared to men.

> **"A poster in all the examining rooms. You know, 'Victims
> of child abuse are welcome.' That's easy. 'Male victims of
> child abuse validated here.' 'We care about the
> victimization of children,' 'Help prevent victimization of
> male children.' Those are messages that you can put on
> posters. 'Let's protect little boys and girls' – see, inclusive.
> Boys and girls who have been victimized as children are
> welcome. *Boys and girls* . . . [and] have the picture – *boy
> and girl*"**[3] (p. 152).

Generally, using patient-centered and gender-sensitive language, and letting individuals know that the clinician is open, non-judgemental, and has an understanding that trauma can affect health can help survivors overcome hesitancy about raising issues pertaining to health. Since the principles of sensitive practice have been developed from survivors' ideas, using them in daily clinical practice should provide a strong indicator of the clinician's awareness of issues of interpersonal violence, and may help counter the feeling of being alone in one's experience of abuse.

One could argue that most of the principles of sensitive practice merely represent good patient-centered care. We suggest that sensitive practice is a "fine tuning" of patient-centered care, a way to ensure that the clinician is aware of the potential effect of interpersonal violence and acts on this awareness with each and every client. Our findings suggest that without adherence to these principles, some survivors will have difficulty tolerating ongoing treatment and perhaps even avoid returning to see the HP.

> "The experience was not beneficial at all. . . . The [clinician] I went to, I felt, was not sensitive at all to the issues of survivors and had no understanding whatsoever about issues that may be a problem to a survivor. And so, I decided that I was just better off avoiding a community [of HPs] that probably was not sensitive to what I was dealing with anyway"[1] (p. 259).

DISCLOSURE OF ABUSE

Disclosure can be a difficult issue for survivor and clinician alike. Some researchers and nurse-midwives argue for the routine screening of all individuals for a history of CSA and other forms of family violence (e.g., Kendall-Tackett, 2004; Seng and Petersen, 1995) and indications of posttraumatic stress disorder (Seng *et al.*, 2002, 2004). Many survivors we spoke with advocated that the clinician take note of behaviors and problems that have been shown to be common in adults who have experienced CSA.

> "But I would ask [HPs] to go a step further, to [talk] . . . to men, particularly males who have addiction problems, who have eating disorders, sleep disorders, depression, anything that has to do with emotion, emotional things or mental health issues. I think it's important that these doctors . . . get trained to be able . . . to identify [behaviors that may be related to past abuse] and to be up on what the actual symptoms are."

The participants in our studies expressed a variety of opinions about whether HPs should routinely ask about a history of CSA.

What is clear from our research is that the participants' opinions on the topic may be seen as existing on a continuum. Participants at one end of this continuum believe that a holistic approach would require all HPs to ask about a history of CSA. One woman said,

> "I think it's important that [HPs] ask questions about abuse as part of a medical history, particularly of women and I think that anyone dealing with women's pain who doesn't ask questions about violence in a woman's life is not doing their job. I feel that very, very strongly"[4] (pp. 92–93).

On the other end of the continuum, participants felt that such inquiries are a violation. This is illustrated by the words of one man, who said,

> "If I wanted to tell him, I'd tell him. It's not his or her business."

Given the evidence that CSA affects health, we think that all HPs should "open the doors to disclosure" (Teram *et al.*, 1999, p. 91) under most circumstances. Our research suggests that there is no one correct way to do so. As participants pointed out, while some survivors may choose to deny a history of CSA, the fact that the question was posed signals that an HP is open to discussion about it. The choice to disclose or not remains with the survivor and will vary with a number of factors including the survivor's perceptions of the HP as trustworthy, whether the survivor feels the inquiry is relevant to his or her health, the level of his or her acknowledgement of the abuse, and his or her stage of healing.

We have identified two types of disclosure (Teram *et al.*, 1999). The first type, termed *task-centered disclosure*, may be initiated by the clinician to seek or, by the client, to provide information specific to an examination or procedure. Task-centered inquiry involves three components: (1) inquiring about discomforts, (2) asking open-ended questions, and (3) remaining alert to body

TABLE 7.1 The three components of task-centered inquiry

Component	Example
1 Inquire about discomforts, sensitivities	"Have you ever had difficulties with an examination of your back?" If answer is yes: "How can I make you feel more comfortable?"
2 Include an open-ended question	"Is there anything else you think I should know before we begin the examination/ procedure?"
3 Repetition of the above	"You seem to become tense whenever I work on your feet. Is there anything I can do differently to make this treatment easier for you?"
	Or
	"And now I would like to move on to examine your feet. Do you have particular discomfort when someone touches your feet?" If answer is yes: "What can we do to make it easier for you?"

language and signs of poor treatment response while using task-centered questions on an ongoing basis (see Table 7.1 for examples). Task-centered inquiry affords the survivor the opportunity to disclose as much information as he or she is comfortable revealing without having to disclose specifics about past abuse.

The second type of disclosure is the explicit sharing of information about past abuse offered spontaneously by the survivor or in response to questions from the HP. The choice to disclose was difficult for most participants because as one woman pointed out,

"Every time you disclose you expose yourself."

Some survivors believe that it is important to inform their health providers about their abuse history because the knowledge helps providers to better understand their health problem and their response to treatment. One woman said,

> **"[disclosure would help the HP to] have some of the understandings of the feelings that are associated with that part of the physical exam, the shame and the guilt and the things that you have going on inside your head. The flashbacks that could happen while you're having an exam. The not being present in the moment."**

For many, the choice to disclose was related to a positive connection they felt with the HP, which led them to expect the HP to respond sensitively to the disclosure. Thus, for many survivors, the process of disclosure involves monitoring the situation and their relationship with the HP, and making decisions about how much information to reveal and when to do so.

Participants urged HPs to "look beneath the surface," to note symptoms that are commonly seen in individuals who have experienced abuse and inquire accordingly. Some expressed the wish that HPs talk to them about the potential health effects of abuse. When asked if he would have welcomed a question about abuse earlier in his life, a man who began dealing with issues regarding sexual abuse in his forties responded by saying,

> **"I've asked myself that a number of times as to would I have been ready to work through that and probably the answer is no. . . . But, I think with opening that door, the process of my working through that stuff and awareness coming to the surface . . . would have been . . . speeded up, yeah. At least I would have felt that possibly it was ok to talk about this."**

The participants in our studies spoke in some detail about how they want a HP to respond to a disclosure of abuse and offered the following recommendations about responding appropriately to a disclosure of CSA.

COMPONENTS OF AN EFFECTIVE RESPONSE TO DISCLOSURE OF PAST ABUSE

ACCEPTANCE OF THE INFORMATION

Survivors said it was very important that the HP communicates that he or she has heard the disclosure and accepts it. One woman described a response to her disclosure that she found very unhelpful:

> "I told the physical therapist about my history of abuse. She didn't acknowledge it. . . . She just kept right on going with what she was doing. . . . Oh boy, if somebody says it, then you've got to acknowledge it. Because then what that says to me is that it's not valid, it's not important, it doesn't have anything to do with us"[4] (p. 95).

AN EXPRESSION OF EMPATHY OR CARING

Another woman gave this example of a positive response of a HP to her disclosure:

> "He just looked at me and he said, you know, 'I'm really sorry this happened to you.' And that was the best thing he could have said."

This simple statement conveys empathy and concern and, followed with a request such as "Tell me how I can help you during your time with me", opens the door to a discussion about what the survivor wants from the HP.

CLARIFY THE LEVEL OF CONFIDENTIALITY

Survivors indicated that they have concerns about information about past abuse being documented in their health care records:

> "Having a written record of my abuse history makes me feel uncomfortable. I may say to a physician – 'I'll tell you but I don't want anything on my record. But if this is between you and I . . .' "

NORMALIZE: ACKNOWLEDGE THE PREVALENCE OF ABUSE

The HP who lets the survivor know that he or she is aware of the startling statistics regarding CSA and that the survivor is not alone is experienced by most survivors as supportive.

VALIDATE THE SURVIVOR'S EXPERIENCE AND THEIR DECISION TO DISCLOSE

Survivors said it was helpful when HPs recognized that it took much courage to disclose a history of CSA. They also felt validated when the HP affirmed that abuse is never the child's fault. In addition, being asked about their sources of support and whether they would like a referral for counseling is also experienced by many survivors as validating. At the same time, survivors advised caution when raising the issue of counseling so as to avoid giving the message that the clinician does not want to deal with abuse issues or that every survivor needs counseling. One man described the following experience with his family doctor:

> "His response was one of understanding and concern. I felt he was concerned. I felt he . . . understood where I was coming from and asked me questions which helped me, little by little disclose more of my deep dark secrets and help me to ask more questions . . . and so when I did see him he was constantly giving me thoughts, ideas, people to contact, how to deal with issues. His wasn't just a one response thing . . . like, if I was coming back in for something else he would ask me how I was doing."

DISCUSS THE IMPLICATIONS OF DISCLOSURE FOR FUTURE INTERACTIONS BETWEEN THE SURVIVORS AND HP

Survivors were quick to point out that they did not expect the clinician to "fix" or take charge of everything for them. One woman said,

> "Don't push the person and be really aware not to use the 'shoulds,' like 'you should call the crisis line' . . . or 'are you seeing a therapist?' "[1] (p. 259).

Indeed, many told us that the reaction from the HP that they hoped for was simply to listen and acknowledge the disclosure. Because disclosure may provoke anxiety and other painful emotions, it is important to offer reassurance and to open a discussion about the client's specific health needs. Invitations such as "Do you have any suggestions about how we could make the examination more comfortable for you?" and "As we proceed, please tell me if I am doing anything that doesn't feel right to you" communicate the HP's willingness to listen and share control. In order to address the vulnerability that a survivor may experience as a result of disclosing, the HP is encouraged to follow up at the next interaction by asking how the client has been since the previous appointment.

SALIENT ISSUES FOR MALE SURVIVORS OF CSA

While many of the long-term sequelae of CSA are similar for men and women (Banyard *et al.*, 2004), our interviews with male survivors revealed that differential gender-based social and cultural contexts may contribute to dissimilar experiences for male survivors when they seek health care. We have reported the male participants' experiences in a recent paper (Teram *et al.*, 2006), and highlight some of the findings here.

Most of the men we interviewed talked about their perceptions that males face barriers to disclosing and resolving a history of CSA not shared by girls and women. They referred to the skepticism about the idea of males being sexually abused (particularly by a woman) that is prevalent in society today; some had experienced this skepticism in interactions with HPs. They pointed out that some people believe that a male who is sexually abused by a woman is "lucky" to have been seduced by an older, more experienced sex partner (Teram *et al.*, 2006). One man said,

"As a child, I told doctors but again nobody would really take it seriously because at that time, to them, it just didn't happen. It may have happened to maybe women or girls or something, but not to boys. That was more or less the general attitude about them. . . . If you were

lucky enough to be raped by a woman then you're lucky.
The side-effects of the experience, this is bad. I was
7 years old but a lot of that was taken away from me,
that young innocence or whatever. I have hidden talents
that I was never able to relive because I've been afraid
of people . . . I was afraid of mostly women"[3]
(pp. 503–504).

Another man described his experience with HPs as one in which
the seriousness of his abuse was minimized:

"Well no, they're not saying, 'I don't believe you.' Some
of them will say to you, 'well you know – sexual
experimenting.' And I told them 'well look, I was sexually
abused by someone who was 18 years old approximately
and I was about 11. There's no sexual experimentation
there, not on my part. I was abused. I wasn't
experimenting. I didn't even know what the hell sex
was.' I think for a lot of doctors it is discounting the
importance of what happened or blaming the victim,
blaming myself. To me that's very damaging when you're
told that"[3] (p. 504).

Men who had been abused by other men talked of how the
stigma and fear associated with homosexuality affected their
own responses to being abused. For some, the abuse led to
uncertainty about their sexual orientation and concern that it
meant that they were homosexual. Many of the men also talked
about their fear that HPs would think they were homosexual if
they revealed their history of CSA.

"This physician here in [name of city], like he says, 'Are
you bisexual?'. . . . Right away to me as a victim he's
stating that I'm bisexual. Like I just wanted to give him a
slap and say, 'Listen you know, I'm not gay'[3] (p. 505).

Another man said,

"You are automatically assumed to be gay and that you
deserved it [the sexual abuse]"[3] (p. 505).

Others, having internalized societal homophobia, talked about how their abuse experiences had led to some strong negative feelings about individuals, including HPs, they perceived to be homosexual. One man said,

> "I had to go into the hospital where I had a problem with some medication I had [taken] and there was a male nurse there and he was obviously very effeminate, and he had to give me an IV. I refused him because I didn't want him touching me"[3] (p. 506).

Male survivors must also deal with the myth that all male survivors are potential perpetrators of CSA. Current research indicates that only a small proportion of males who are sexually abused go on to abuse others and that many male perpetrators do not report a history of CSA (Glasser *et al.*, 2001; Lambie *et al.*, 2002; Salter *et al.*, 2003). Despite this, however, misconceptions remain. One man said,

> "I felt like I was an abuser. I was part of it or I was going to become an abuser because I had been abused. I felt dirty. I was scared. I was confused. I didn't know anything about anything. All I knew was how ugly I felt inside and all the problems I had"[3] (pp. 507–508).

Male participants also talked about how society's stereotypes of men and manliness add another layer of difficulty for male survivors:

> "We [men] all have been taught that we've got to be strong and we've got to be in control and be the 'he man' and have the armor and be strong when we don't feel that way at all, we feel the opposite, especially male survivors."

Many of the men talked about how this image of what a man should be led them to deny that they had been abused and contributed to their great reluctance to seek help when they could no longer deny that they had been harmed.

One participant spoke of his need for HPs to use what he termed *malecentric communication* (Teram *et al.*, 2006). He said,

> "Malecentric type of messages with no shame. Okay? We recognize that mental health is a serious issue and we care for men in this community. This is a safe harbor for you; we welcome you. That's the way you need to talk"[3] (p. 512).

Few studies have examined HPs' attitudes towards and practices with male survivors of CSA, but studies of mental health professionals (Day *et al.*, 2003; Lab *et al.*, 2000) indicate that most underestimate the prevalence of CSA in males, few have specific training or experience working with male survivors, and few routinely ask men about a history of CSA (Holmes and Offen, 1996; Lab *et al.*, 2000). Given this lack of awareness among mental health professionals, it is highly probable that HPs oriented toward the body are also unaware of the issues salient to male CSA survivors (Teram *et al.*, 2006). The second edition of the *Handbook on Sensitive Practice* will strongly encourage HPs to recognize the prevalence rates of childhood sexual abuse of boys, consider their own biases, and promote environments and practices that will be more accepting and supportive to male survivors of CSA. The second edition of the *Handbook* (Schachter *et al.*, in press) will be available on the Public Health Agency of Canada's National Clearinghouse on Family Violence website in Fall 2008.

THE INTERSECTION OF RACE, CULTURE, ETHNICITY, AND CSA

Our ability to comment on how race, ethnicity, and culture may impact interactions between survivors and HPs is limited because most participants were Caucasian. However, the words of the eight Aboriginal participants have reinforced that culture powerfully affects the meaning and experience of illness and the response to treatment. One Aboriginal woman said,

> "I went to a massage therapist and I had a medicine bundle on and she took it off and people aren't supposed to touch that, so I thought she was kind of

uneducated about Aboriginal beliefs but even that is a boundary you don't just go up to someone and take their jewellery off them. It's pretty personal. She took it off and I told her, 'I don't like taking it off, can I have it back on?' And she said, 'No, I can't massage you with it on. you have to keep it off.' And I didn't feel comfortable after that. The massage didn't even help."

Every HP should be respectful of cultural beliefs and practices, and participate in an ongoing, active process to learn more about the cultures and worldviews of the clients with whom they work (see e.g., Waxler-Morrison *et al.*, 2005).

WHAT DOES SENSITIVE PRACTICE LOOK LIKE?

In order to illustrate the principles of sensitive practice, the working groups of survivors and HPs outlined specific and detailed guidelines for clinicians. Space does not permit us to discuss all of these recommendations, but we offer the following as some salient examples.

CREATING AND MAINTAINING A SENSITIVE ENVIRONMENT
Survivors emphasized that creating a safe environment depends on all individuals in a health-serving environment (including support and administrative personnel) understanding the dynamics of interpersonal violence and following the principles of sensitive practice. For example, the widespread practice of having the receptionist inquire about the nature of the problem when booking appointments is problematic for many survivors. The working groups suggested that in order to determine how long an appointment to book, receptionists might ask, "Is the visit for discussion or an examination?" This approach demonstrates respect for clients' boundaries in terms of privacy.

CLOTHING
Many HPs do not appreciate the difficulty that undressing and wearing an examination gown causes for some individuals. One man said,

"If I had to take off clothing . . . for a male doctor it's . . .
hard because there's the trust issue there and for me
there was a lot of guilt and shame . . . I struggle with
body image and sometimes . . . I feel powerless then."

Survivors said that having the HP negotiate clothing options so as
to allow clients to wear undergarments whenever possible or
encouraging clients to dress in clothing that facilitates
examining/procedures (e.g., shorts, bathing suits) demonstrates
respect for the client and willingness to share control. The
working groups also suggested that HPs provide gowns in a
variety of sizes and/or shorts, avoid the use of paper gowns and
sheets, and minimize the length of time that a client is
undressed. One woman said,

"He was probably one of the most sensitive people I've
encountered. I was really surprised. First of all, I kept my
underwear on but he still had me wrap myself in one of
the paper sheets, and was very careful in terms of how
he handled me . . . in his case it was a case of him saying
'Could you turn so I could just look at your back, I need to
see this spot in particular.' So, it left me in control of me
and my person. So I was really, I was very impressed with
that."

PREPARING THE CLIENT FOR AN APPOINTMENT,
TREATMENT OR HOSPITAL STAY
Providing information about health care processes before an
appointment, treatment, or hospital admission is very helpful in
reducing the client's anxiety and a key principle of sensitive
practice. Written information can be sent to clients before the
first appointment or given to them to read as they wait. Respect
and fostering a mutual learning process involves making sure
that the reading level of all printed material is such that most
clients can understand it (around grade 6 to grade 8 level). Even
when printed resources are supplied, it is still important to
explain the procedures verbally and ensure that the client has

understood, especially if English is not the client's first language or if he or she has reading problems. An example of such preparatory information is included in the *Handbook* (Schachter *et al.*, in press).

THE INITIAL MEETING

NEGOTIATING ROLES AND ENCOURAGING THE PRESENCE OF A SUPPORT PERSON

Sharing control means that HPs invite a discussion of roles and expectations early in the initial contact. This provides the client with an opportunity to request clarification or communicate any discomfort, and therefore facilitates a two-way exchange of information. When a HP communicates a willingness to have a client-chosen support person in the consulting room with the client, she or he demonstrates respect and understanding of the vulnerability which many clients feel. Such communication also directly contributes to a sense of safety. One man said,

"I can remember feeling awkward about having another man touch me. But my wife was right beside me too, she was in the room anyway and it was easier. I felt safer."

A caveat about including a support person is to ensure that the needs of the client are paramount. For instance, since spousal abuse is typically masked for public appearances, HPs should meet briefly with the client alone and ask if he or she wants the support person present during the session. This communicates that the clinician is aware of and knowledgeable about interpersonal abuse.

GENERAL SUGGESTIONS FOR THE INITIAL MEETING

The following suggestions emerged from the working groups of survivors and clinicians. The principle of sensitive practice that it reflects is included in brackets.

- Do not assume that the client knows what the HP is going to do or the reason for his or her actions (*share information*). One woman told us,

"I found quite often when you go to a doctor or physiotherapist, they automatically assume that you have some kind of knowledge of their job outline. . . . And why should I know? I didn't go to school for that, so it's really frustrating. And they expect you to know something about it"[1] (p. 255).

- Take the health history before asking the client to remove any clothing (*respect for boundaries*).
- Because many survivors have learned to ignore their bodies, take enough time for the client to answer questions and describe symptoms during the health history (*respect and fostering a mutual learning process*).
- Seek a balance between offering descriptors of symptoms ("Would you describe the pain as sharp or dull, throbbing or aching?") and encourage the survivor to "own" his or her symptoms by describing them in his/her own words (*fostering a mutual learning process*).
- If the client appears to be uncomfortable or is having difficulty responding to one aspect of the assessment, move on to another part of the assessment and return to the previous questions later (*respect and understanding that healing is not a linear process*).
- Use a written informed consent that has been drafted in "client-friendly" terms. Let the client know that consent can be withdrawn at any time without reprisal (*share control*).
- Ensure privacy for undressing and dressing, and confirm that the client is ready by knocking, asking permission, and *waiting for permission* before entering the room (*respect for boundaries*).
- Explain what is involved and the rationale for each segment of the objective and subjective evaluation (*share information*).

SUGGESTIONS REGARDING THE OBJECTIVE PHYSICAL
EXAMINATION

- Ask for verbal consent before proceeding with each segment
  of the examination (*share control*). One man said,

  > "Information, and knowing just before you're going to
  > be touched that it is coming, so it wasn't sort of a
  > shock to you that you were being touched."

- Approach the examination as an opportunity to teach the
  individual about his or her body and symptoms (e.g., referred
  pain) (*foster a mutual learning process*).

- Ensure that the client clearly understands that he or she can
  ask you to pause, slow down, or stop the physical exam (*share
  control, taking time*).

- Emphasize that you are willing to be flexible during the
  evaluation and subsequent treatment to reduce the client's
  discomfort or anxiety (*respect for boundaries*). One woman
  reported,

  > "I had been seeing her for six months. I kept
  > postponing my physical and the MD noticed that. She
  > kept bringing it up and reminding me until I finally
  > told her that I was frightened of laying flat on my back
  > in a paper gown. She told me that it would not be a
  > problem for me to be partially sitting up throughout
  > the whole examination including the pelvic exam. Now
  > she tells all of her patients that that is an option. She
  > told me that it had been an important conversation for
  > her."

- Inquire intermittently about the client's well-being and his or
  her willingness to continue, especially when shifting the exam
  from one part of the body to another or if the client
  communicates discomfort or distress. This may be done in
  various ways. For example, an HP could say, "I am going to
  touch your back, is that okay?" or "How are you doing?"
  "Can we continue?" If the individual indicates that he or she
  cannot continue, the HP should stop what they are doing and
  talk through the situation before proceeding (*share control*).

■ *After the examination, see the client, at least briefly, in a fully-dressed state. This acknowledges the client as a whole and equal person (respect).*

These suggestions may mean that an initial evaluation takes longer than anticipated or may need to be carried out over two appointments. Taking extra time may help establish rapport, trust, and safety and often saves time in the long run.

WHAT TO DO IN MOMENTS OF UNCERTAINTY: SAVE THE SITUATION

In spite of efforts to practice sensitively, all clinicians experience occasions when they are uncertain about what the client is experiencing, or they become aware that the client is upset. The working groups suggested actions that fit the mnemonic **SAVE** to remind HPs to *Stop, Appreciate, Validate, and Explore.* This is offered as a general guide for any difficult situation

TABLE 7.2 SAVE – a mnemonic for health professionals when dealing with difficult or confusing situations

Stop	Stop what you are doing, recognizing this as a moment of difficulty that touches both the client and clinician.
Appreciate	Use the helping skill of immediacy. Share your observations and invite the client to tell you what is happening for her or him (e.g., "You look very uncomfortable. Can you tell me what is happening (how you are feeling)?") If client does not respond, "Can you tell me what will help? or What you need? or What I can do to help you?"
Validate	Validate and empathize with the client (e.g., "Don't worry" or "This can be difficult").
Explore	Once the client is able to continue, negotiate your own and the client's actions for the remainder of the interaction. Discuss the implications for future interactions and health care as appropriate.

including periods when clients become tearful or experience strong emotions, or when the HP suspects that the client may be experiencing a dissociative episode or flashback. Table 7.2 above provides examples.

SELF-CARE AND RECOGNIZING THAT HPS CAN ALSO BE SURVIVORS

We have urged HPs to recognize that hearing about abuse experiences from clients is distressing for most people (Schachter *et al.*, 2001). We have also encouraged them to extend the compassion they have for their clients to themselves, and to seek support when working with a client who reports a history of CSA. Working closely with individuals who have experienced trauma and hearing about their experiences can lead to distress for any HP. The effects vary depending on the individual, but may include symptoms that are similar to PTSD: intrusive thoughts, nightmares, depersonalization. This response has several labels including secondary traumatic stress, compassion fatigue (Figley, 1995), and vicarious traumatization (VT; McCann and Pearlman, 1990; Saakvitne and Pearlman, 1996). McCann and Pearlman argue that VT is a normal response which results from empathizing with traumatized clients. The negative effects can be minimized by awareness of the reality of VT and attention to ways that individuals and organizations can anticipate and address it (Saakvitne and Pearlman, 1996).

It is also important to remember that survivors of CSA and health professionals are not two discrete groups. A significant proportion of HPs are themselves survivors of CSA (Kendall-Tackett, 2004). A HP who has a personal history of CSA may be able to be especially empathic towards survivors of abuse, particularly if he or she has worked through his or her own reactions and has healed the wounds associated with the abuse. For some, it may be more difficult to hear the experiences of clients who are suffering deeply. All clinicians need to give themselves permission to talk with a trusted colleague about their reactions (without breaching the client's confidentiality). If these emotional responses are not processed, they can lead a clinician to avoid survivors or unintentionally communicate that the client has done something wrong. Being a highly skilled helper does not preclude the need for support and assistance for oneself.

CONCLUSION

Findings from our own studies and from those reported elsewhere in this book demonstrate that abusive and traumatic experiences affect health in many ways. In addition to symptoms of psychological distress and negative effects on an individual's physiology, trauma can impede the individual's ability to interact with HPs and/or to tolerate health care examinations and procedures. By virtue of their specialized education and greater social power, clinicians have an ethical responsibility to maximize the benefits of the health care experience and to do no harm. Survivors in our studies emphasized that HPs' insensitivity can trigger the perception of danger in the client-clinician encounter and *can do harm*. In some instances, this harm is retraumatizing and adds to the individual's burden, decreasing the probability that he or she will benefit from the current or future treatment.

It is also incumbent on mental health professionals to recognize the important role they can play in facilitating productive interactions between their survivor clients and other HPs (Stalker *et al.*, 1999). Counsellors, therapists, and other mental health professionals can help survivors to recognize when a history of abuse is negatively affecting their ability to access and/or make constructive use of health care services. They can assist their clients with developing strategies to overcome barriers and to communicate more effectively with their health care providers, and when necessary, they can advocate directly with HPs on behalf of their clients and their needs. Many abuse survivors would benefit from efforts by mental health and physical health professionals to collaborate for their benefit. When mental and physical health professionals work together, we are more likely to overcome the problems inherent in a health care system that separates the body from the mind (Kendall-Tackett, 2004).

Client-centered practice views individuals as whole human beings, and focuses on body and mind, on physical, emotional, and spiritual needs, and on how the individual's family, work, culture, position in the life cycle and other contextual factors all affect the experience of illness and the experience of help-seeking (Brown *et al.*, 1999). Sensitive practice may be seen as a tool to enhance client-centered care to ensure that the spectrum of effects of CSA on health is in the forefront of the clinician's mind and actions when working with every client.

NOTES

1 From "Toward sensitive practice: Issues for physical therapists working with survivors of childhood sexual abuse" by C.L. Schachter, C.A. Stalker, and E. Teram (1999). *Physical Therapy, 79*. Copyright 1999 by American Physical Therapy Association Inc. Reprinted with permission.

2 From *Handbook on sensitive practice for health professionals: Lessons from women survivors of childhood sexual abuse* by C.L. Schachter, C.A. Stalker, and E. Teram (2001). Ottawa: Health Canada. Copyright 2001 by Health Canada. Reprinted with permission.

3 Copyright (2006) From "Towards malecentric communication: Sensitizing health professionals to the realities of male childhood sexual abuse survivors" by E. Teram, C.L. Schachter, C.A. Stalker, A. Hovey, and G. Lasiuk. *Issues in Mental Health Nursing, 27*, 499–517. Reproduced by permission of Taylor & Francis Group, LLC, http://www.taylorandfrancis.com.

4 From "Opening the doors to disclosure: Childhood sexual abuse survivors reflect on telling physical therapists about their trauma" by E. Teram, C.L. Schachter, and C.A. Stalker (1999). *Physiotherapy, 85*, 88–97. Copyright 1999 by Elsevier Limited. Reprinted with permission.

REFERENCES

Arnow, B.A., Hart, S., Scott, C., Dea, R., O'Connell, L., and Taylor, C.B. (1999). Childhood sexual abuse, psychological distress and medical use among women. *Psychosomatic Medicine, 61*, 762–770.

Banyard, V.L., Williams, L.M., and Siegel, J.A. (2004). Childhood sexual abuse: A gender perspective on context and consequences. *Child Maltreatment, 9*(3), 223–238.

Brown, J.B., Stewart, M., and McWilliam, C.L. (1999). Using the patient-centered method to achieve excellence in care for women with breast cancer. *Patient Education and Counseling, 38*(2), 121–129.

Day, A., Thurlow, K., and Woolliscroft, J. (2003). Working with childhood sexual abuse: A survey of mental health professionals. *Child Abuse and Neglect, 27*(2), 191–198.

Felitti, V.J. (1991). Long-term medical consequences of incest, rape, and molestation. *Southern Medical Journal, 84*(3), 328–331.

Felitti, V.J., Anda, R.F., Nordenberg, D., Williamson, D.F., Spitz, A.M., Edwards, V., Koss, M.P., and Marks, J.S. (1998). Relationship of childhood abuse and household dysfunction to many of the leading causes of death in adults. *American Journal of Preventive Medicine, 14*, 245–258.

Fergusson, D.M., and Mullen, P.E. (1999). *Childhood sexual abuse: An evidence based perspective*. Thousand Oaks, CA: Sage

Figley, C. R. (ed.) (1995). *Compassion fatigue: Coping with secondary traumatic stress disorder in those who treat the traumatized*. New York: Brunner/Mazel.

Finkelhor, D. (1990). Early and long-term effects of childhood sexual abuse: An update. *Professional Psychology: Research and Practice, 21*, 325–330.

Finkelhor, D. (1994a). The international epidemiology of child sexual abuse. *Child Abuse and Neglect, 18*(5), 409–417.

Finkelhor, D. (1994b). Current information on the scope and nature of child sexual abuse in the community. *The Future of Children, 4*(2), 31–53.

Glaser, B., and Strauss, A. (1967). *The discovery of grounded theory*. Chicago, IL: Aldine.

Glasser, M., Kolvin, I., Campbell, D., Glasser, A., Leitch, I., and Farrelly, S. (2001). Cycle of child sexual abuse: Links between being a victim and becoming a perpetrator. *British Journal of Psychiatry, 179*, 482–494.

Harrop-Griffiths, J., Katon, W., Walker, E., Holm, L., Russo, J., and Hickok, L. (1988). The association between chronic pelvic pain, psychiatric diagnoses and childhood sexual abuse. *Obstetrics and Gynecology, 71*, 589–594.

Holmes, G., and Offen, L. (1996). Clinicians' hypotheses regarding clients' problems: Are they less likely to hypothesize sexual abuse in male compared to female clients? *Child Abuse and Neglect, 20*(6), 493–501.

Hulme, P. (2000). Symptomatology and health care utilization of women primary care patients who experienced childhood sexual abuse. *Child Abuse and Neglect, 24*(11), 1471–1484.

Kendall-Tackett, K. (2002). The health effects of childhood abuse: Four pathways by which abuse can influence health. *Child Abuse and Neglect, 26*, 715–729.

Kendall-Tackett, K.A. (2004). Epilogue: Where do we go from here? In K.A. Kendall-Tackett (ed.), *Health consequences of abuse in the family: A clinical guide for evidence-based practice* (pp. 247–251). Washington, DC: American Psychological Association.

Lab, D.D., Feigenbaum, J.D., and De Silva, P. (2000). Mental health professionals' attitudes and practices towards male childhood sexual abuse. *Child Abuse and Neglect, 24*(3), 391–409.

Lambie, I., Seymour, F., Lee, A., and Adams, P. (2002). Resiliency in the victim-offender cycle in male sexual abuse. *Sexual Abuse: A Journal of Research and Treatment, 14*(1), 31–48.

Lampe, A., Solder, E., Ennemoser, A., Schubert, C., Rumpold, G., and Sollner, W. (2000). Chronic pelvic pain and previous sexual abuse. *Obstetrics and Gynecology, 96*(6), 929–933.

Lesserman, J., Li, Z., Drossman, D.A., and Hu, Y.J.B. (1998). Selected symptoms associated with sexual and physical abuse history among female patients with gastrointestinal disorders: The impact on subsequent health care visits. *Psychological Medicine, 28*, 417–425.

Levin, M., and Greenwood, D. (2001). Pragmatic action research and the struggle to transform universities into learning communities. In P. Reason and H. Bradbury (eds), *Handbook of action research* (pp. 103–113). London: Sage.

Little, P., Everitt, H., Williamson, I., Warner, G., Moore, M., Gould, C., *et al.* (2001). Obervational study of effect of patient centredness and positive approach on outcomes of general practice consultations. *British Medical Journal, 323*, 908–911.

McCann, I.L., and Pearlman, L. (1990). A framework for understanding the psychological effects of working with victims. *Journal of Traumatic Stress, 3*, 131–149.

Monahan, K., and Forgash, C. (2000). Enhancing the health care experiences of adult female survivors of childhood sexual abuse. *Women and Health, 30*(4), 27–41.

Newman, M.G., Clayton, L., Zuellig, A., Cashman, L., Arnow, B., Dea, R., and Taylor, C.B. (2000). The relationship of childhood sexual abuse and depression with somatic symptoms and medical utilization. *Psychological Medicine, 30*, 1063–1077.

Powers, P.H., Goldstein, C., Plank, G., Thomas, K., and Conkright, L. (2000). The value of patient- and family-centered care. *American Journal of Nursing, 100*(5), 84–88.

Project of the ABIM Foundation, ACP-ASIM Foundation, and European Federation of Internal Medicine (2002). Medical professionalism in the new millennium: A physician charter. *Annals of Internal Medicine, 136*, 243–246.

Reason, P., and Bradbury, H. (eds) (2001). *Handbook of action research*. London: Sage.

Reiter, R.C., and Gambone, J.C. (1990). Demographic and history variables in women with idiopathic chronic pelvic pain. *Obstetrics and Gynecology, 75*, 428–432.

Romans, S., Belaise, C., Martin, J. Morris, E., and Raffi, A. (2002). Childhood abuse and later medical disorders in women: An epidemiological study. *Psychotherapy and Psychosomatics, 71*, 141–150.

Saakvitne, K.W., and Pearlman, L. (1996). *Transforming the pain: A workbook on vicarious traumatization*. New York: W.W. Norton.

Safran, D.G., Taira, D.A., Rogers, W.H., Kosinski, M., Ware, J.E., and Tarlov, A.V. (1998). Linking primary care performance to outcomes of care. *Journal of Family Practice, 47*(3), 213–220.

Salter, D., McMillan, D., Richards, M., Talbot, T., Hodges, J., Bentovim, A., *et al.* (2003). Development of sexually abusive behaviour in sexually victimised males: A longitudinal study. *The Lancet, 361*(9356), 471–476.

Schachter, C.L., Stalker, C.A., and Teram, E. (1999). Toward sensitive practice: Issues for physical therapists working with childhood sexual abuse survivors. *Physical Therapy, 79*(3), 248–261.

Schachter, C.L., Stalker, C.A., and Teram, E. (2001). *Handbook on sensitive practice for health professionals: Lessons from women survivors of childhood sexual abuse*. Ottawa, ON: Health Canada.

Schachter, C.L., Teram, E., and Stalker, C.A. (2004). Integrating grounded theory and action research to develop sensitive practice with survivors of childhood sexual abuse. In K.W. Hammell and C. Carpenter (eds), *Qualitative research in evidence-based rehabilitation* (pp. 77–88). Edinburgh: Harcourt.

Schachter, C.L., Stalker, C.A., Teram, E., Lasiuk, G.C., Danilkewich, D. (in press). *Handbook on sensitive practice: Lessons from adult survivors of childhood sexual abuse.* Ottawa, Public Health Agency of Canada.

Seng, J.S., and Peterson, B.A. (1995). Incorporating routine screening for history of childhood sexual abuse into well-woman and maternity care. *Journal of Nurse-Midwifery, 40,* 26–30.

Seng, J.S., Sparbel, K.J.H., Low, L.K., and Killion, C. (2002). Abuse-related posttraumatic stress and desired maternity care practices: Women's perspectives. *Journal of Midwifery and Women's Health, 47,* 360–370.

Seng, J.S., Low, L.K., Sparbel, K.J.H., and Killion, C. (2004). Abuse-related post-traumatic stress during the childbearing years. *Journal of Advanced Nursing, 46*(6), 604–613.

Sickel, A.E., Noll, J.G., Moore, P.J., Putnam, F., and Trickett, P.K. (2002). The long-term physical health and healthcare utilization of women who were sexually abused as children. *Journal of Health Psychology, 7,* 583–597.

Stalker, C.A., Schachter, C.L., and Teram, E. (1999). Facilitating effective relationships between survivors of childhood sexual abuse and health professionals. *Affilia: Journal of Women and Social Work, 14*(2), 176–198.

Stalker, C.A., Carruthers-Russell, B.D., Teram, E., and Schachter, C.L. (2005). Providing dental care to survivors of childhood sexual abuse. Treatment considerations for the practitioner. *The Journal of the American Dental Association, 136,* 1277–1281.

Stewart, M. (1995). Effective physician-patient communication and health outcomes: A review. *Canadian Medical Association Journal, 152*(9), 1423–1433.

Stewart, M. (2001). Towards a global definition of patient centered care. *British Medical Journal, 322,* 444–445.

Stewart, M., Brown, J.B., Weston, W.W., McWhinney, I.R., McWilliam, C.L., and Freeman, T.R. (1995). *Patient-centered medicine: Transforming the clinical method.* Thousand Oaks, CA: Sage.

Stewart, M., Brown, J. B., Weston, W.W., McWhinney, I.R., McWilliam, C.L., and Freeman, T.R. (2003). *Patient-centered medicine: Transforming the clinical method.* Abingdon, UK: Radcliffe Publishing.

Stewart, M.J., Brown, J.B., Donner, A., McWhinney, O.C., Oates, J., Weston, W.W., and Jordan, J. (2001). The impact of patient-centered care on outcomes. *Journal of Family Practice, 49*(9), 796–804.

Teram, E., Schachter, C.L., and Stalker, C.A. (1999). Opening the doors to disclosure: Childhood sexual abuse survivors reflect on telling physical therapists about their trauma. *Physiotherapy, 85*(2), 88–97.

Teram, E., Schachter, C.L., Stalker, C.A., Hovey, A., and Lasiuk, G. (2006). Towards malecentric communication: Sensitizing health professionals to the realities of male childhood sexual abuse survivors. *Issues in Mental Health Nursing, 27*, 499–512.

Thompson, M.P., Arias, I., Basile, K.C., and Desai, S. (2002). The association between childhood physical and sexual victimization and health problems in adulthood in a nationally representative sample of women. *Journal of Interpersonal Violence, 17*(10), 1115–1129.

Walker, E.A., Katon, W.J., Roy-Byrne, P.P., Jemelka, R.P., and Russo, J. (1993). Histories of sexual victimization in patients with irritable bowel syndrome or inflammatory bowel disease. *American Journal of Psychiatry, 150,* 1502–1506.

Walker, E.A., Katon, W., Harrop-Griffiths, J., Holm, L., Russo, J., and Hickok, L.R. (1988). Relationship of chronic pelvic pain to psychiatric diagnoses and childood sexual abuse. *American Journal of Psychiatry, 145,* 75–80.

Walker, E.A., Gelfand, A., Katon, W.J., Koss, M.P., Von Korff, M., Bernstein, D., and Russo, J. (1999a). Adult health status of women with histories of childhood abuse and neglect. *American Journal of Medicine, 107*(4), 332–339.

Walker, E.A., Unutzer, J., Rutter, C., Gelfand, A., Saunders, K., VonKorff, M., et al. (1999b). Costs of health care use by women HMO members with a history of childhood abuse and neglect. *Archives of General Psychiatry, 56*(7), 609–613.

Waxler-Morrison, N., Richardson, E., Anderson, J., and Chambers, N.A. (eds) (2005). *Cross-cultural caring: A handbook for health professionals* (2nd edn). Vancouver, BC: UBC Press.

Yehuda, R. (2001). The biology of posttraumatic stress disorder. *Journal of Clinical Psychiatry, 62* (suppl. 17), 41–46.

8

Health care can change from within

A sustainable model for intimate partner violence intervention and prevention

Bruce Ambuel, Mary Beth Phelan, L. Kevin Hamberger, and Marie Wolff

---

INTIMATE PARTNER VIOLENCE (IPV) is now recognized as a common and significant source of morbidity and mortality worldwide. The impact falls most directly and severely on women as a result of multiple mechanisms including intentional injury from physical assault, deprivation, neglect, psychiatric morbidity, and stress-related illness. However, children and other family members are often direct and second-hand victims of intimate partner violence. Both direct and second-hand exposure to IPV are associated with an increased risk of illness during the period of exposure, and for years after the person has escaped the violent environment. Because of these health consequences, many professional organizations now recognize that physicians, nurses, and other health care professionals have an important role to play in identifying victims of IPV, intervening to help victims of IPV, and ultimately preventing IPV.

This has not always been the case – health systems have not historically recognized IPV as a health care problem. Even today, health care providers frequently fail to address IPV as a health issue, identify IPV victims, or offer appropriate primary and secondary prevention services. Health care clinics often fail to incorporate the techniques of systems-based practice, continuous quality improvement, and networking with community resources to support the clinician's efforts regarding IPV. The health care culture often fails to communicate values and norms supporting women's equality and respect, opposing violence against women as well as other forms of interpersonal violence, and supporting abuse victims.

Much research since 1990 has focused upon improving the health care response to IPV. We now know that professional education will improve practitioners' knowledge, attitudes, and clinical skills. We also know that changes in clinic policies, procedures, and quality improvement processes will lead to temporary improvements in clinical care provided to victims of IPV. However, no studies have demonstrated comprehensive, sustained improvement in the health care response to IPV.

Our goal is to design an intervention model that creates sustainable change in the health care response to intimate partner violence. The model we describe builds upon elements of previously successful educational and systems change interventions targeting health care providers and health care clinics. These successful components are integrated into an intervention model designed specifically to address sustainability by *changing the culture of the medical clinic and health care organizations* so that IPV intervention and prevention is institutionalized.

BACKGROUND

THE DEFINITION AND DYNAMICS OF IPV
Our work in designing and implementing a sustainable health care-based model of IPV prevention and intervention has been guided by the following working definitions. *Interpersonal violence* is the threatened or actual use of physical force or

power against another person, which causes, or has a high likelihood of causing, deprivation, injury, or death (World Health Organization, 1996). *Intimate partner violence* (IPV), or *domestic violence*, is violence that occurs between two people who currently or in the past shared an intimate relationship such as marriage, a non-marital partnership, or a dating relationship. IPV is a chronic, long-term problem in a relationship. The abusive party, or batterer, will use various acts of power and violence to control, punish, and dominate their partner. Mechanisms of IPV include physical assault, unwanted sexual contact, destruction of property, harm to pets, harm to friends or family, stalking, and psychological terror. The type and pattern of violence typically varies over time, as the abuser relies upon physical assault on one occasion, forced sex on another, and dehumanizing and controlling behavior on another.

The psychological terror which occurs in an abusive relationship deserves some specific discussion because the intensity of this abuse can be difficult for many people to understand. Psychological terror tactics are used intentionally and systematically to destroy social networks by prohibiting contact with others, humiliating the person in front of friends, family, and co-workers, or directly threatening others. A potent element of psychological abuse is a constant barrage of disparaging and degrading comments made in the privacy of the home. A final element of psychological terror is the fact that it occurs in the context of other types of violence including life- and health-threatening physical and sexual assault. The totality of the abuse leaves the victim feeling helpless, hopeless, worthless, constantly vigilant, and always vulnerable to assault. Psychological terror includes controlling *when* the person may leave the home, *where* they may go, and with *whom* they may speak. The batterer often controls when and where the person sleeps, when and what they eat, when they may visit a physician, and when they may fill prescriptions and take medication.

THE IMPACT OF INTIMATE PARTNER VIOLENCE ON HEALTH

Intimate partner violence is a social and medical epidemic that adversely affects the physical and emotional well-being of victims (Coker et al., 2002; Hamberger and Phelan, 2004). The medical consequences are numerous, including injury and its associated short- and long-term disability (Beck et al., 1996; Coben et al., 1999; Hartzell et al., 1996; Le et al., 2001; Perciaccante et al., 1999), death (Rennison and Welshers, 2000), poorer self-reported health (Cascardi et al., 1992; Wagner and Mongan, 1998), posttraumatic stress disorder (PTSD), substance abuse disorders (Cascardi et al., 1992; Kyriacou et al., 1999), depression (Saunders et al., 1993), anxiety disorders (Gleason, 1993), and suicide (Stark and Flitcraft, 1995). In fact, women who experience IPV have more health problems and hospitalizations *for all causes* than women who have not experienced IPV (Bergman and Brismar, 1991). The medical consequences of IPV are dire, and victims of IPV regularly seek medical care yet are infrequently detected by physicians (Rath et al., 1989; Hamberger et al., 1992; Rodriguez et al., 1999).

THE PRIMARY CARE CLINIC EMERGENCY DEPARTMENT AS ENTRY POINT

These health consequences have obvious implications for primary care clinics serving adults. Screening for IPV is also important in pediatric settings (American Academy of Pediatrics, 1998). Studies have shown that between 30 percent and 59 percent of women with children who are abused admit to experiencing battering within an intimate relationship (Campbell, 1994; McKibben et al., 1989; Stark and Flitcraft, 1988). In addition to the direct trauma children may incur during disputes, child witnesses of domestic violence have been shown to be at risk for developmental delay, sleep disorders, school failure, oppositional defiant disorder, depression, and child abuse (Edleson, 2000).

The emergency department is also an important point of entry into the health care system for persons experiencing domestic violence. The 24-hour availability of health care allows for any patient to be evaluated for any problem, regardless of payer status. Usually, a patient–physician relationship has not been previously established, resulting in an anonymous evaluation of sensitive issues such as domestic violence. This set of conditions, combined with the fact that nationally, partner violence results in at least 1.4 million emergency department visits annually (Muelleman *et al.*, 1998), places the emergency department in a unique position to screen, perhaps the most vulnerable persons, for domestic violence.

A study by Muelleman and Liewer (1998) suggests that the emergency department is also well positioned for the early detection and prevention of IPV. They found that a cohort of women who initially visited an emergency department without an IPV-related complaint presented to the emergency department with an IPV-related complaint at the same rate as a cohort of women who initially presented to the emergency department with IPV. The follow-up period in their study was five years. This research suggests that women presenting to emergency departments are a high-risk population.

IPV AND HEALTH DISPARITIES
IPV is a direct cause of health disparities – women who are experiencing or have experienced IPV are more likely to seek health care episodically for acute problems and less likely to seek preventive health care (Johnson and Elliott, 1997). In addition, although IPV is a significant cause of morbidity and mortality across all socioeconomic groups, women are at higher risk of IPV when they are poor, young, socially isolated, developmentally delayed, or experiencing chronic mental illness. Therefore IPV contributes to the documented health disparities experienced by these most vulnerable groups of women.

IPV IN WISCONSIN
Regional and local statistics help to illustrate the true social consequences of IPV as well as the impact on women's health and well-being. Consider the state of Wisconsin as an example,

the location of the authors' parent institution, the Medical College of Wisconsin. *Healthiest Wisconsin 2010* (Wisconsin Department of Health and Family Services) identifies intentional injuries and violence as one of 11 top health priorities for the state. As noted above, IPV is a major cause of intentional injury for women. In addition, exposure to IPV increases a woman's risk in four other *Healthiest Wisconsin* priority areas: alcohol, substance abuse and addiction; mental disorders; high-risk sexual behaviors; and access to primary and preventive health services.

Intimate partner violence is the most common cause of intentional injury for women in the State of Wisconsin and in southeastern Wisconsin. In 2002, there were 38 IPV homicide victims in Wisconsin, accounting for half of the female homicides that year. A majority of these IPV homicides occurred in southeastern Wisconsin including 14 in Milwaukee County, and five in neighboring Waukesha County. Domestic violence advocates in the Milwaukee County District Attorneys' office worked with 4,978 victims of IPV in 2003 while the Waukesha County District Attorneys worked with 1,184 victims. The City of Waukesha, a jurisdiction of only 65,000 people, reported dispatching 789 domestic violence-related police calls in 2003.

Not surprisingly, the local IPV prevention agencies in Milwaukee and Waukesha County serve a large number of clients who are victims of IPV. In 2003, Sojourner Truth House, one of three shelters in Milwaukee County, fielded 15,964 phone calls to their hotline, provided 10,558 nights of shelter to 713 women and children, and treated 601 men in their batterers treatment program. The Women's Center, Inc., the sole shelter in Waukesha County, fielded 6,005 crisis calls and provided 6,146 nights of emergency shelter to women and their children. The Women's Center provided face-to-face services to 827 adult victims of domestic violence and their 255 children including emergency shelter, individual and group counseling, and personal and legal advocacy for battered women and their children.

Regarding incidence and prevalence in Wisconsin health care settings, a classic 1992 study by Hamberger *et al.* (1992) showed that 25 percent of women in a family medicine clinic in southeastern Wisconsin had experienced IPV in the past year. This figure is consistent with numerous subsequent studies conducted in many geographic locations, in which observed rates of current IPV among women seeking primary care services has ranged from 17 percent to 32 percent. A recent study by Kramer and colleagues (2004) provides an excellent snapshot of the community based upon a survey of 1,268 women presenting to 24 emergency departments and primary care clinics affiliated with one health care system in eastern Wisconsin. Women in this study reported a 50 percent to 57 percent lifetime prevalence of physical and/or emotional abuse, and a 26 percent prevalence of sexual abuse. When asked about the past year, 6 percent reported severe physical abuse, 12 percent physical abuse, 4 percent sexual abuse, and 28 percent emotional abuse. Only 25 percent had *ever* been asked about IPV, yet 86 percent indicated that they would disclose abuse if asked "directly, respectfully, and confidentially." Particularly significantly, abused women reported lower health status than non-abused women, suggesting that exposure to IPV is a hidden source of morbidity in this diverse population of women.

THE HEALTH CARE RESPONSE TO IPV

In recognition of the profound medical and social consequences of IPV, many professional organizations recommend that physicians, clinics, and hospitals take systematic steps to identify victims of IPV, intervene appropriately to assist the patient, and document results and plans in the medical record (American Academy of Pediatrics, 1998; American College of Emergency Physicians, 1995, 2002; American College of Obstetricians and Gynecologists, 1995; American Medical Association, 1992). These recommendations include: asking patients about current exposure to IPV; taking a history of past interpersonal violence including IPV, child physical and sexual abuse, sexual assault, stalking, and emotional abuse; offering appropriate intervention and referral, depending upon the patient's history;

documentation in the medical record; and patient education and prevention.

These professional recommendations are supported by research that has explored the treatment preferences of female patients in general, and battered women specifically (Hamberger *et al.*, 1998; Rodriguez *et al.*, 1996). Women expect physicians to ask patients about IPV. They expect physicians to provide effective and compassionate health care for battered women who present with injury or illness. They expect physicians to ask victims of IPV about the safety of children in the home, offer support, for example, by stating that the violence is not the victim's fault and that they have a right to be respected and safe, assist in safety planning, make referrals to community resources, and express concern regarding safety when the physician believes a woman is in a dangerous situation.

SCREENING FOR IPV IN HEALTH SETTINGS

Although women want physicians to take an active role in IPV identification, intervention, and prevention, there has been limited empirical evidence that the health status of women will improve when primary care physicians screen for IPV, identify victims, and provide prevention and intervention services. However, recent studies suggest that health care interventions, including IPV screening and referral, have a positive effect on patients' lives (Krasnoff and Moscati, 2002; McFarlane *et al.*, 2006). In 2006, McFarlane *et al.* reported on a cohort of 360 women identified in a primary care setting as experiencing IPV. The researchers used a randomized, two-armed clinical trial to compare two interventions for women experiencing IPV. Participants' safety behaviors, use of community resources, and levels of violence following one of two interventions were assessed over a two-year period. The two interventions tested were a wallet-sized referral card with community resources and recommended safety behaviors, or a 20-minute nurse case management protocol. The nurse case manager intervention included reviewing a validated set of safety behaviors, empathetic listening, anticipatory guidance with respect to the legal system, shelter use or counseling as well as referrals tailored to the patient's situation, such as shelter or job training. Estimated time for the intervention was 20 minutes. Participants were assessed every six months and evaluated for the following measures: threats of assault, actual assault, danger risks for homicide, work harassment, safety behaviors, and community resource use. Irrespective of the intervention group, all women experienced a statistically significant reduction in threats of abuse, physical abuse, workplace harassment, and danger assessment, suggesting that a simple assessment and advocacy benefits abused women.

Emergency departments, family medicine, and pediatrics clinics have considerable potential to function as violence prevention centers that offer universal screening, assessment, and medical treatment of injuries and illnesses related to domestic violence, interventions, provision of safety planning, legal advocacy and risk assessment and documentation (Dutton *et al.*, 1996). Further, emergency departments and primary care clinics can potentially play important roles in providing professional and community education with respect to IPV (Hamberger and Phelan, 2004).

A key unanswered question is how to improve the health care response to IPV. Various attempts to improve physician and health clinic responses to IPV have been only marginally successful. Despite the link between IPV and negative health outcomes for women and their children, and despite recommendations for universal screening, many physicians do not routinely screen for IPV (Rodriguez *et al.*, 1999), and many clinics do not provide sufficient organizational support for IPV identification and prevention (McCleer *et al.*, 1989). Health care clinics that have attempted to improve the response to IPV have either failed to improve care, or struggled to achieve only modest improvement in patient care. The responsibility for ensuring an effective response to IPV within the health care system cannot lie solely with individual physicians or nurses. Assuring quality care for victims of IPV is a responsibility shared by the entire clinic health care team and health care organization.

A number of studies have begun to illuminate challenges that must be overcome to create a sustained improvement in the care provided to battered women. The challenges identified to date fall into two broad categories: health care providers, and health care clinics and organizations.

HEALTH CARE PROVIDERS

At the individual level, physicians, nurses, and other clinicians may not identify and assist victims of IPV for a variety of reasons (Hamberger and Patel, 2004; Sugg and Innui, 1992). Many clinicians simply do not recognize that IPV is a problem that needs to be addressed in their practice, either because they do not believe that IPV is a legitimate health care problem, or because they dramatically underestimate the prevalence in their own practice and the community where they practice. Clinicians who recognize IPV as a problem often avoid asking patients about it because they report that they lack the knowledge, training, and clinical experience to incorporate IPV identification and prevention into their routine practice. Some clinicians perceive that they do not have time to identify and help abused patients – a perception that certainly interacts with lack of knowledge and experience and with lack of support from the clinic system (discussed below).

Fear is yet another reason why clinicians avoid asking patients about IPV. Some clinicians fear that they will offend patients if they ask about IPV (a fear contradicted by research). Other clinicians fear that they will place themselves and employees in their practice at risk if they identify and attempt to help victims of IPV in their practice. A final barrier that physicians report is lack of knowledge about community resources to which they may refer victims of IPV.

Although physicians face many barriers to IPV intervention, several studies have identified factors that facilitate IPV intervention. Sugg and Innui (1992) found that physicians were more likely to screen if they had an experience early on in their career helping a patient who was a victim of IPV, or if they personally knew someone who was a victim of IPV. Rodriguez *et al*. (1999) reports that female physicians are more likely to routinely screen patients for IPV than male physicians, and that male physicians working in a clinic with female physicians are more likely to screen for IPV than male physicians working by themselves or in a clinic with other male physicians.

HEALTH CARE CLINICS AND ORGANIZATIONS

A number of studies have attempted to improve the health care response to IPV by training clinicians *and* implementing changes in the clinic operations. The mixed results of these studies are instructive. Harwell *et al*. (1998) implemented the RADAR training model in 12 community health centers to increase IPV screening, identification, and referral. Clinicians' knowledge and comfort (measured at baseline, after training, and after three months) increased following training, but declined to baseline at the three-month follow-up. Chart audits in four clinics showed that the rate of screening increased, and safety assessment increased, but documentation of abuse did not change.

Fanslow *et al*. (1998, 1999) compared IPV care in two emergency departments, one control and one intervention where staff received IPV training. The intervention clinic was no different from the control in identification of patients experiencing IPV. Within the intervention clinic, there was a modest increase in the number of confirmed cases of IPV and in interventions offered. However, these increases were not maintained at a one year follow-up.

Thompson *et al*. (2000) conducted an intensive, one-year intervention to improve asking about DV, case finding, and management in primary care using a group-randomized control trial with five primary care clinics. Outcome measures included a baseline and follow-up survey of clinicians and medical record review. Among clinicians, self-efficacy increased while fear of offending the patient and fear of jeopardizing staff safety decreased. Documentation of screening increased by 14 percent, but case finding did not increase. The clinics' use of routine patient health questionnaires containing IPV questions accounted for virtually all the increase in identification. Display of IPV posters for patients was also important.

Campbell *et al.* (2001) studied 12 hospital emergency departments in Pensylvania and California that were randomized into intervention and control conditions. Staff from the intervention condition participated in IPV training. Staff in the experimental condition scored higher in staff knowledge and IPV attitudes, and higher in patient satisfaction. However, there was no difference between the intervention and control condition in identification of IPV in the medical record.

McCaw *et al.* (2001) implemented one of the broader IPV interventions using multiple strategies including physician training, patient education posters and brochures, environmental prompts for clinicians, clinician feedback on referrals to support identification, referral to on-site resources for assistance, and connections to a local IPV agency. The authors' report increased clinician referral and patient self-referral to the on-site IPV counselor, increase patient self-report of being asked by clinicians about IPV, and increased patient satisfaction with the clinic's approach to IPV.

Hamberger *et al.* (2004) provided a three-hour IPV training program to 752 nurses and mental health clinicians working in various departments within a hospital (behavioral health; emergency department; endoscopy; obstetrics and gynecology, and women and infants) as part of a health system's strategy of improving care for victims of IPV. Following training, these clinics were asked to implement IPV-identification-and-intervention protocols. Focus groups were then conducted to assess the response of each clinic (Minsky-Kelly *et al.*, 2005). They identified a number of significant barriers including questions about appropriateness and value of universal screening for certain patient categories, inadequate provider expertise, and concern about time and workload. A particularly important finding of

Minsky-Kelly *et al.* is that each of the clinics encountered some barriers that were unique to that clinic environment. For example, obstetrics and women and infants clinics encountered a conflict between the value of family-centered care and the value of screening patients for IPV in private, and the emergency department worked with many non-English-speaking patients who have a different cultural background. Another significant barrier was that some physician groups were not interested in IPV.

CHANGING HEALTH CARE CULTURE

We can draw several conclusions from this group of studies that have attempted to improve the health care system response to IPV. First, at the level of the individual clinician, training that focuses upon knowledge, attitudes, and clinical skills is essential but not sufficient for creating sustained changes in clinical care. Second, at the level of the clinic and health system, systems-change strategies are also essential but not sufficient for sustained change in clinical care of IPV victims. Helpful strategies are patient questionnaires that include IPV history, chart prompts and chart tools, quality improvement methods with feedback to clinicians, and patient education through posters, brochures, and clinician discussion. Third, there are many barriers to creating sustained improvement in the quality of IPV identification, treatment, and prevention. As Minsky-Kelly *et al.* (2005) discovered, some of these barriers are predictable from the literature, but some are unique to specific settings and to specific groups of clinicians. It is likely that some of these barriers cannot be anticipated in advance, but are rooted in cultural norms and must be discovered and overcome as part of the change process.

We believe that sustained improvement in the health care response to IPV requires a cultural change such that primary and secondary prevention of IPV is supported by the clinic's and health system's prevailing values, norms, and staff roles. Interventions which rely only upon clinician training or systems improvement will not produce sustained change. We have designed the *Health Care Can Change from Within* intervention model to address all three elements necessary for sustained improvement in the primary and secondary prevention of IPV: clinician training, health system change, and cultural change.

HEALTH CARE CAN CHANGE FROM WITHIN: A MODEL FOR SUSTAINED IMPROVEMENT IN IPV PREVENTION

INTRODUCTION

The model we are implementing, Health Care Can Change From Within, seeks to effect change at multiple levels, including changing knowledge, attitudes, clinical skills, and clinical behavior of health care providers and their administrative support, changing clinical policies and procedures to support these individual behavioral changes, and thereby creating self-sustaining improvement in the system response of the medical clinics to IPV. The ultimate goal is improving the health of women by creating a system-wide response to partner violence prevention. Five key objectives of this model are:

1 Recruiting select staff from each clinic to receive intensive, in-depth training in IPV – these *health care advocates* will become leaders of the clinic's response to IPV.

2 Training all physicians, clinical, and administrative staff in relevant knowledge, attitudes, and behavioral skills relevant to their role.

3 Facilitating change in clinic systems, including implementing strategies for primary and secondary prevention of IPV, creating clinical and administrative policies and procedures, and implementing continuous quality improvement to monitor and improve the system response.

4 Creating change in the clinic culture, including roles, norms and values, which sustain improvement over time.

5 Creating a partnership between the health care clinic and local community-based nonprofit organizations that work on intimate partner violence and family violence.

THE IMPORTANCE OF SELF-CARE

Self-care is an essential element of all training programs that address IPV (Ambuel *et al.*, 1997, 2003). Because interpersonal violence is so prevalent in our society, participants in any educational program will include people who have experienced intimate partner violence, sexual assault, child abuse, dating violence, workplace violence, or other forms of interpersonal violence. Many staff members will know a friend or relative who is in an abusive relationship or has experienced violence. Some people, who have never experienced any type of violence, will find the content of training upsetting because of the dreadful and repugnant nature of family violence and partner violence. For this reason every training program needs to have an intentional strategy to address self-care (Ambuel *et al.*, 1997). In the Change from Within model, the issue of self-care is addressed in each training session by discussing the issue and letting participants know that they are free to excuse themselves from part of the training if they feel that participation would be traumatic. Participants are also told that they may step out of the room if needed during the training. Participants are reminded of resources that are available locally such as support groups, the human resources department, advocacy agencies, employee assistance programs, counseling, and so on.

Facilitators and supervisors should be aware that training in intimate partner violence will sometimes raise issues of workplace violence and abuse because the dynamics of workplace violence and abuse, particularly in health care educational and clinical settings, are often similar to the dynamics of intimate partner violence (Warshaw, 1996). Supervisors should be prepared to respond sensitively and effectively to concerns about workplace abuse and violence. Some clinics have entrenched problems with workplace violence that may include psychological abuse, sexual harassment, or other types of interpersonal violence. It is difficult, if not impossible, to implement the Change from Within model in a work setting where interpersonal workplace violence is systemic and condoned implicitly or explicitly. Therefore these issues need to be addressed and resolved prior to training.

OBJECTIVE 1: TRAINING HEALTH CARE ADVOCATES
Health care advocates are an innovative and essential element of the Change from Within model. Each clinic that implements the model begins by recruiting two or more staff members who participate in an intensive 20-hour training program on IPV and health care. These staff members will become on-site *health care advocates* who will be responsible for leading the clinic's response to IPV. One of their first roles will be to support the training of other clinical and office staff in IPV prevention. After other clinic staff members have been trained (see Objective 2), the health care advocates will support and guide the clinics' implementation of primary and secondary prevention of intimate partner violence. The primary prevention methods may include selecting, displaying, and distributing patient education materials about IPV and healthy relationships. Primary prevention may extend to brief counseling provided by physicians and/or nurses regarding healthy relationships. Secondary prevention may include the design and implementation of clinical protocols for physicians, nurses, and other staff to identify patients who are current or past victims of IPV and intervene. Because the health care advocates will be recognized for their training and expertise, other staff will approach them for advice and consultation regarding patients who are experiencing IPV. From time to time, the advocate may also work directly with a patient who is in crisis.

The health care advocates will also serve as a resource for clinic committees and administrators as they develop or revise policies and procedures, and implement continuous quality improvement initiatives to monitor clinical outcomes related to IPV prevention and seek improvement. Of particular importance, the health advocates' roles and responsibilities will be integrated into the advocates' job description so that the clinic makes an organizational commitment to their leadership role, which continues into the future.

OBJECTIVE 2: TRAINING PHYSICIANS AND OTHER CLINIC STAFF MEMBERS

Once health care advocates have been trained, they help organize training programs for physicians, other clinical staff, and administrative staff in their clinic. Experienced educators in IPV facilitate these trainings. All clinical and administrative staff – physicians, nurses, physician assistants, medical assistants, lab and x-ray technicians, other clinical staff, reception, scheduling, billing, and other administrative staff – participate in training on the primary and secondary prevention of IPV. This training covers knowledge, attitudes, and behavioral skills relevant to their respective roles in the clinic. Physicians receive four hours of training, while administrative staff members receive three hours of training. Nursing and other clinical staff members participate in either a three- or four-hour training, depending upon the clinic's choice.

The training program for physicians is based on Ambuel *et al.*'s Family Peace Project curriculum (1997). This training begins with what we call *Intimate Partner Violence 101*, basic information on the definitions and interpersonal dynamics of intimate partner violence, as well as common misunderstandings. This portion includes a learning activity, which introduces participants to the personal voices and biographies of survivors, either through a small group discussion with one or two community mentors (survivors of IPV; Ambuel *et al.*, 1997), or by viewing a video interview with survivors, such as *Voices of survivors* by Nicolaides (1999).

Physicians are introduced to the concepts of primary and secondary prevention of intimate partner violence. Primary prevention means interventions directed at adults and adolescents who have not experienced IPV with the goal of imparting knowledge and behavioral skills that *immunize* them against IPV. This includes understanding the characteristics of a healthy relationship, understanding the characteristics of abusive behavior and abusive relationships, and developing the skills to establish effective boundaries in relationships. Secondary prevention refers to identifying people who are victims of IPV and intervening to provide support. The goal is to reduce the impact of IPV by identifying and assisting victims/survivors early in the course of the problem, and/or helping victims/survivors make changes so that they achieve safety in their interpersonal relationships.

Physician training also reviews the impact of IPV on an individual patient's health and upon the health care system, the recommended health care response to IPV (including primary prevention, identification, intervention, documentation, follow-up, and awareness of community resources). Physicians receive specific coaching in and opportunities to practice clinical skills for patient interviewing related to secondary prevention. This practice addresses many of the most common concerns of physicians: How do I ask patients about IPV? Will I offend patients if I ask? What do I do when a patient says yes? How do I document accurately, effectively, and efficiently? Can I do anything that truly helps a woman in an abusive relationship? How do I deal with the most complex presentations such as a patient with an apparently intentional injury who insists the injury was accidental, or a potentially abusive partner who is reluctant to leave an exam room? What are my ethical and legal obligations?

Physician training includes a component on the health clinic's system response. This is essential because one cannot expect physicians to sustain new clinical practices unless they receive appropriate support from the rest of the staff and the work environment, such as participation of others in screening, appropriate chart tools, patient education materials, patient questionnaires, and other resources. The systems-based clinic changes will include implementation of routine IPV prevention, screening and intervention, display of educational posters and brochures that address IPV prevention, staff training, changes in clinic policies and procedures, and other systems-level strategies that support IPV prevention.

The syllabus for training non-physician staff members is similar to that used with the physician training. However, it is adapted to the roles, behavioral skills, and social and environmental factors relevant to each staff member's work setting in the clinic. For example, while nurses, physician assistants, and medical assistants may receive training in interviewing that is similar to physician training, reception staff will receive training focused on interacting with patients in public areas of the clinic or on the telephone, and relaying observations to nurses and physicians.

The syllabus for training in educational settings, such as medical school or medical residency clinics, includes an educational component – how to teach the clinical skills necessary to identify and help victims and survivors of IPV. Two elements are of particular importance. First, how to productively engage learners to explore personal values and attitudes regarding partner violence, as well as the sociological and cultural context of violence against women. Second, how to teach interviewing skills in real time in clinical settings.

Trainees in our intervention model are not passive consumers of new information about partner violence. All clinic staff members are expected to participate as a team in leading system change and improvement. To encourage broad participation in this change process, our training programs engage the participants in a dialogue about strengths and weaknesses in the clinic's current response to IPV. As an outcome of this dialogue, each work area in the clinic is expected to identify strengths and weaknesses in the clinic's current response to IPV, as well as a list of things to *keep doing, stop doing* and *start doing* in order to improve the team's response. This leads us into the next objective of the intervention model – creating sustained improvement in the clinic system.

OBJECTIVE 3: CLINICAL SYSTEMS CHANGE
Primary care clinics and emergency departments are complex organizations where staff members often fulfill multiple roles with competing demands upon their time. The workload fluctuates depending on disease and injury trends in the larger

community, placing a premium upon efficiency during periods of peak workload. In addition, the knowledge and regulatory environment in health care changes rapidly, requiring constant change in clinical protocols and clinic operations. Within these layers of complexity, physicians, nurses, and other staff work to provide the best possible care to each individual patient. Because the environment is so complex, one cannot expect physicians, nurses, or other staff to implement and sustain changes in clinical care unless there are also corresponding changes in the clinic system which allow them to do so efficiently and effectively. A team approach is required in which all team members have similar expectations and expect similar outcomes, and where the clinic system – workflows, policies, and procedures – is organized to achieve and sustain these outcomes.

Clinics that implement the Change from Within model are asked to make many changes – large and small – to enhance their system response to intimate partner violence. These changes address primary and secondary prevention of intimate partner violence, continuing education for professional and office staff, use of continuous quality improvement strategies to measure change, and development of written policies and procedures. The Change from Within model outlines general goals and guidelines for system's change, but each clinic is expected to apply these general guidelines and engineer their own local solution that meets local needs.

SECONDARY PREVENTION

Secondary prevention is the centerpiece of the health system response to intimate partner violence. The centerpiece of secondary prevention is identifying current and past victims/survivors of IPV. Therefore, each clinic is expected to implement systems to identify, assess, and help patients who are current or past victims of intimate partner violence, including routine screening of specific patient groups to identify IPV using validated questions on patient health history questionnaires or validated interview questionnaires asked by nurses and clinicians as part of the history-taking process. Each clinic also implements case-finding protocols to assess for IPV any patient who presents with possible intentional injury, or with a pattern of non-specific physical or psychological signs and symptoms that may be caused by stress and psychological abuse. Brochures and posters that encourage patients to talk with their physician if they have concerns about IPV can supplement screening and case-finding protocols.

Once a patient has been identified as a current or past survivor of IPV, the clinic is expected to provide emotional support; to further assess the patient's history and current circumstances, including risk of further injury or death; and offer appropriate interventions including safety planning, referral to community resources, referral to shelter, engagement of on-site resources (social work), patient education materials, and so on. As a final step in secondary prevention, the physician and nurse are expected to document the visit in the patient's medical record using chart templates such as body maps and structured notes to enhance the medical record.

PRIMARY PREVENTION

The Change from Within model considers primary prevention – building competence and resilience through patient education about healthy relationships – as an essential element of a comprehensive clinical response to IPV; therefore each clinic will devise a patient education strategy that covers healthy relationships as well as stalking, dating violence, sexual assault and partner violence. The target audience for primary prevention is broad, including adolescent girls and boys, adult women, and adult men. The total clinic environment may be used for education by taking full advantage of brochures, posters, pictures, newsletters, magazines, web pages, e-mail communication, and so on. Although the Change from Within program provides various resources for patient education, each clinic is expected to devise their own education strategy geared towards their facility and patient population.

CONTINUING EDUCATION

An essential component of sustainability is fostering growth of knowledge and skills among administrative and clinical staff. Fortunately there is a strong tradition of continuing education in health care settings that our intervention can build upon. As described above, the initial Change from Within intervention includes an extensive training for health care advocates, and intensive basic training for all other administrative and clinical staff, with a goal of training 80 percent of each group. To sustain the level of staff education and interest, each clinic is expected to establish a protocol for training those personnel who cannot attend the basic training, for training newly hired staff, for providing an annual continuing education program on IPV, and for encouraging those interested to seek additional training.

CONTINUOUS QUALITY IMPROVEMENT

Continuous quality improvement (CQI) is a well-accepted method within health care for defining, measuring, and improving clinical outcomes, and sustaining these improvements. Each clinic implementing the Change from Within model therefore implements a continuous quality improvement process to establish clinical outcomes, measure success in achieving these outcomes, and revise the intervention to achieve further improvements. The CQI process begins with an assessment of strengths and gaps in the clinic's current response to IPV. The clinic staff can then identify locally determined clinical outcomes for improvement. For each clinical outcome identified for improvement, the clinic staff must identify specific, measurable clinical indicators. These indicators are then monitored over time, with feedback provided collectively and to individual practitioners. The specific clinical objectives and indicators are determined locally by the clinic staff in response to their own assessment of strengths and gaps, and their understanding of the needs of their local population. Local control also allows the professional clinicians to respond and adapt to changes in our knowledge base as new literature is published.

WRITTEN POLICIES AND PROCEDURES

An organization's written policies and procedures are a formal declaration of their intended goals and methods of practice. Clinics implementing the Change from Within model are expected to incorporate these various changes in practice into written policies and procedures. Revising existing policies related to IPV, or drafting new policies may accomplish this. These policies describe in some detail the protocols for primary prevention, secondary prevention, continuing education, patient education, and continuous quality improvement. These policies also describe the responsibilities and goals of each staff member in the clinic regarding IPV prevention, the flow of communication among staff members, who and how information is documented, and workflow.

OBJECTIVE 4: CHANGING THE CLINIC CULTURE

What do we mean by changing a clinic's *culture* regarding intimate partner violence prevention? We use the term *culture*, in the context of a medical clinic, to refer to the *values, norms*, and *material culture* of the clinic which are sustained over a period of days, weeks, months, and years. *Values* are ideas one has about what is important in life, or, in the specific context of the medical clinic, what is important within the work life of the clinic. Cultural values relevant to the Change from Within model include the following: (1) that IPV is a health care problem because it is a significant and preventable cause of morbidity and mortality due to intentional injury; (2) that medical clinics can provide a haven for victims of intentional injury where they may receive healing, education, and support; and (3) that physicians, nurses, and other clinic staff have important roles to play in helping to prevent IPV.

Norms are expectations of how people will behave in different situations, or in the context of the medical clinic, how various employees will behave in different situations in the workplace. Norms go hand-in-hand with formal and informal methods of social control that maintain norms through positive or negative social feedback. The cultural norms relevant to the Change from Within model include the expectation that each person working in the clinic, including clinical and administrative staff, can play an important role in a systematic, team-approach IPV prevention, that clinical staff can identify victims of IPV, offer help and document appropriately in the medical record, and that all employees have a role to play in creating a supportive, respectful, and healing environment.

Material culture refers to the physical things which are manifestations of values and norms. Examples of material objects, in the context of the medical clinic, include the medical record that organizes information in a specific format for the physician; the health history form completed by a new patient before seeing the physician; artwork and patient education posters on the walls; and even the physical layout of the reception area, waiting room, and exam rooms. Some examples of material culture relevant to the Change from Within model include mechanisms in the medical records to prompt nurses and physicians to ask patients about IPV, patient education brochures and posters on healthy relationships, partner violence, or safety planning, and even the clinic's written policies and procedures regarding IPV.

The concept of culture implies continuity over time. The Change from Within model has been designed intentionally to produce sustained changes in values, norms, and material culture of medical clinics. Some of the strategies we have adopted to facilitate sustained change in clinic culture include:

1 **Creation of the health advocate role, which embodies values supportive of IPV prevention. The presence of the health advocate is intended to support these values in the clinic workplace, and to help create new norms and the feedback processes to sustain these norms.**

2 **Comprehensive training of all staff in a short period of time is intended to create momentum for making and sustaining changes in clinical practice.**

3 The Change from Within model emphasizes local decision-making and control of specific elements of the intervention. In a sense, the Change from Within model is a *tool-box* of ideas, concepts, model policies, and procedures, medical records tools, questionnaires, patient education hand-outs, posters, CQI methods, and other tools that clinic staff can use to implement effective IPV prevention. This allows clinic staff to adapt the intervention to local assets and needs of the clinic and patient population, and simultaneously builds local ownership and investment in the change process.

4 The Change from Within model uses two accepted methods of institutional change in health care settings – creation of policies and procedures coupled with continuous quality improvement to integrate changes into medical culture.

5 A final factor that will help sustain the cultural change is provider satisfaction with patient response. We expect that patients will respond positively to physicians, nurses, and other clinic staff as they implement primary and secondary prevention efforts. In addition, some patients in desperate, abusive relationships will be identified and receive support. These clinic outcomes will help reinforce the clinical changes.

OBJECTIVE 5: BUILDING TRUE PARTNERSHIPS WITH LOCAL WOMEN'S ADVOCACY AGENCIES

True community partnership and collaboration are fundamental to the Change from Within model (Hamberger and Ambuel, 2000). Partners include the health care clinic, local nonprofit women's advocacy organization, and health care professionals with expertise in IPV prevention. Each of these partners contributes essential knowledge and skills to help the clinic reach the goal of sustainable change.

The health care clinic makes a commitment to undertake all elements of the intervention program described above, including recruiting health care advocates, organizing training for clinical and administrative staff, revising or implementing policies and procedures, making environmental changes, providing ongoing staff training, and implementing quality improvement processes. The women's advocacy agency develops expertise in the Change from Within model, trains health care advocates, participates in training clinic staff, and provides ongoing support to the clinic, primarily through the health advocates. Local violence prevention experts support the training of health advocates and clinic staff run the training programs for clinical professionals – physicians, nurses, physician assistants, medical assistants – and advise the clinic regarding quality improvement and program evaluation.

The Change from Within model incorporates four facets of partnership and collaboration.

ADAPTATION TO LOCAL CONDITIONS AND INSTITUTIONAL NORMS

Some elements of the Change from Within model are well described in the program training manuals. However, other elements are intentionally left vague because staff at the health clinic and women's advocacy organization are expected to adapt the intervention to meet local community needs and institutional norms.

SHARED ROLES

All partners share multiple roles while implementing the Change from Within model. These include adapting the training program for the individual needs of clinic staff, developing primary prevention strategies suited for the clinic's patient population, integrating screening and intervention protocols and tools into the clinic work flow and medical records system, designing ecologically valid evaluation methods that answer questions relevant to the local clinic and advocacy agency, and disseminating knowledge and experience gained from the intervention.

MUTUAL RESPONSIBILITY

All partners make a commitment to provide timely and respectful feedback to each other throughout the partnership, share leadership roles, and protect the safety and rights of patients and clinic staff. An important symbol and tool for assuring mutual responsibility is the explicit discussion of partnership, and the drafting of partnership agreements that describe roles, responsibilities, and processes for resolving misunderstandings or problems. Each partner designates one liaison to the project who will be responsible for resolving problems that inevitably arise.

MUTUAL BENEFIT

Partners make a commitment to each other to assure that the intervention is mutually beneficial at the outset, and continues to be mutually beneficial. Some of the benefits are directly related to the project's intended outcomes. For example, the collaboration should increase partners' knowledge, skills, and credibility for interventions in health care systems, increase staff skill and professionalism, and increase the safety and health of women and children. In addition, the partners should achieve indirect benefits such as supporting staff professional development and discovering opportunities for future collaboration.

EVALUATING THE CHANGE FROM WITHIN MODEL

The Change from Within model must be evaluated at three levels of analysis: individual change in clinicians and clinic staff, change in the health care clinic system, and cultural change. Of course, the ultimate test of the model will be improvement in the health, safety, and well-being of female patients and others exposed to IPV. We expect that physicians will show a demonstrable improvement in behavioral skills in carrying out IPV prevention tasks, as well as an increase in IPV attitudes and knowledge. Clinics are expected to show *sustained improvements* in various areas including: (1) written policies and procedures that describe the clinic's planned response to IPV; (2) patient education through posters, brochures, and discussion; (3) use of clinical protocols for prevention, screening, intervention, and documentation; (4) chart tools, such as body injury maps, interview chart prompts, and patient health surveys that will support efficient work by physicians and nurses; and (5) evaluation of clinical indicators with feedback to clinicians on their individual performance. Evaluation of cultural change and sustainability will require the development of new measurement strategies.

EXPERIENCE TO DATE

At the end of our first year implementing the Change from Within model with four clinics, two family medicine, one pediatrics and one emergency department affiliated with the Medical College of Wisconsin, we have learned a number of lessons regarding implementation.

COLLABORATION TAKES TIME

Developing and implementing an intervention that involves three partners (health clinics; IPV clinical experts; and IPV advocacy agencies) is a time- and labor-intensive endeavor. The initial step is to obtain buy-in from key leaders. The recruitment of health advocates must be guided by criteria that facilitate the effectiveness of the project and may take several months to ensure that the most qualified staff are identified for this critical role. Scheduling the training of health care advocates can be a logistical challenge. Time for training must be scheduled in the midst of busy schedules at multiple agencies. Training in emergency departments presents additional, unique challenges because they operate 24 hours a day, seven days a week, have relatively large staffs, and require training of multiple shifts of personnel.

Changing clinic systems to actively support the primary and secondary prevention of IPV is a slow and incremental process. Organizational policies and procedures have to be revised, clinical protocols and chart prompts for screening, case finding, referral and medical record documentation have to be developed or revised, quality assurance measures have to be put in place, outcomes determined, indicators established, and continuing education expectations developed. Essentially, the effort is aimed at changing clinical practice, which is a process that takes time, repetition, and feedback regarding results. Clinics are responsible for changing their clinic environment by ensuring that brochures, posters, and other educational materials are readily available in the clinic. These educational materials have to be culturally and literacy appropriate for the setting, and even such issues as placement of materials may have to be negotiated among clinic staff.

Culture change does not happen quickly or without some difficulty. The intent of this intervention is to dramatically change the norms and values of the clinic so that the primary and secondary prevention of IPV is seen as a key objective in the clinics' health care delivery. If respected opinion leaders embrace this culture change, it will be disseminated and adopted more easily by other staff.

INVOLVEMENT OF COMMUNITY PARTNERS AND CLINICAL IPV EXPERTS FROM THE BEGINNING

The community agencies and clinical IPV experts have shared responsibility for implementing the Change from Within model from the beginning. Both groups have participated in designing and implementing the intervention. Faculty and community partners meet monthly and are in frequent e-mail and telephone contact between meetings. All aspects of the intervention have received input from both community and academic partners, including the development and implementation of the training as well as system and culture changes.

To develop effective partnerships between community experts and health care providers also takes time. Although both partners typically have the same goals (i.e., preventing IPV and ensuring the safety and well-being of victims), it must be acknowledged that they frequently approach the problem from quite different perspectives (Hamberger and Ambuel, 2000). Thus, a major task in the development of an effective partnership is the development of competency for working with each respective professional and clinical culture, together with the development of trust. We have found that the most important strategy for accomplishing cultural competency and trust is clear and transparent communication. Differences must be addressed with respect for the respective views of the partners. Conflicts must be confronted with openness, willingness to listen, and from the perspective that, ultimately, both parties wish to accomplish the same things. Flexibility and willingness to understand the limitations within which each partner works, and to find solutions that fit within such parameters is necessary. Thus it is important to focus on interests, not positions, and to identify options that facilitate mutual gain, rather than adopt a "win-lose" perspective. Finally, it is important to identify objective criteria for decision-making, leading to mutual decisions and choices.

COMMUNITY AND ACADEMIC SETTINGS ARE DYNAMIC
The IPV intervention takes place within organizational structures that are constantly evolving. Being sensitive to these changes that may impact the effectiveness of the intervention and having the ability to respond and adapt to these changes is required. Changes in leadership, faculty, and staff could all potentially have an effect on the implementation of the model Health Care Can Change From Within. Gaining initial buy-in from leaders is essential, but nurturing and sustaining that buy-in as organizational leadership and priorities shift is equally critical. A close and continual dialogue with all the partners ensures that the intervention model is implemented to ensure maximum success.

SUMMARY
Efforts to improve the health care system's response to IPV have generally met with limited success. We know, for example, that

education can improve physician knowledge, clinical skills training can improve physician clinical skills, use of clinical protocols can improve the consistency of IPV interventions, and IPV screening and brief advocacy can improve the health of women. However, implementing and sustaining these improvements has been a problem. No study to date has demonstrated sustained improvement in the quality of clinical care provided to IPV victims, and several studies show that there can be significant organizational barriers to improved care. The intervention paradigms used in this prior work may be one of the problems, because these paradigms have treated the health care system as a "black box." That is, training is provided to individual health care providers (the input), and evaluation measures changes in screening, identification and intervention with abuse victims (the output). When the training intervention produces short-lived improvements in care which dissipate, this is interpreted as a failure to change the behavior of health care providers. This black box paradigm has been ineffective because it does not take into account the organizational and cultural aspect of the health care systems when designing and evaluating the intervention.

With *Health Care Can Change from Within*, we are proposing an intervention paradigm that opens the organizational black box by striving to make and measure changes in the system of care which will support and complement changes in individual provider knowledge, attitudes, skills and behavior. A critical element of this intervention model is creating change from within the health care system, rather than from outside, by training selected staff members as health care advocates, training all staff who have contact with patients, and asking clinics to use the typical tools of the health care system – policies, procedures, clinical protocols, continuous quality improvement – to improve IPV identification, treatment and prevention. Success in this organizational arena would be reflected in the development of a clinic environment that communicates, through posters, patient education and patient–staff interaction, the clinic's values about violence prevention and healthy relationships. A second critical element of this intervention is establishing and maintaining collaborative relationships with community organizations working on the prevention of family violence. The ultimate measure of the success of the *Health Care Can Change from Within* model is sustained improvements in the quality of IPV identification, treatment and prevention, and improvements in the health and well being of female patients who are at-risk or victims of IPV. Our research team is currently conducting research to evaluate both outcomes.

REFERENCES

Ambuel, B., Hamberger, L.K., and Lahti, J.L. (1997). The Family Peace Project: A model for training health care professionals to identify, treat and prevent partner violence. In L.K. Hamberger, S. Burge, A. Graham, and A. Costa (eds), *Violence issues for health care educators and providers* (pp. 55–81). Binghamton, NY: Haworth Press,

Ambuel, B., Butler, D., Hamberger, L.K., Lawrence, S., and Guse, C. (2003). Female and male medical students' exposure to violence: Impact on well-being and perceived capacity to help battered women. *Journal of Comparative Family Studies, 34*, 113–135.

American Academy of Pediatrics Committee on Child Abuse and Neglect (1998). The role of the pediatrician in recognizing and intervening on behalf of abused women. *Pediatrics, 101*, 1091–1092.

American College of Emergency Physicians (ACEP) (1995). Emergency medicine and domestic violence. *Annals of Emergency Medicine 25*, 442–443.

American College of Emergency Physicians Board of Directors (2002). Emergency medicine and domestic violence. Accessed 4/2004 at www.acep.org.

American College of Obstetricians and Gynecologists (ACOG) (1995). Domestic violence. ACOG Technical Bulletin No. 209. *Journal of Gynecology and Obstetrics 51*, 161–179.

American Medical Association, Council on Scientific Affairs (1992). Violence against women: Relevance for medical practitioners. *Journal of the American Medical Association, 267*, 3184–3195.

Beck, S.R., Freitag, S.K., and Singer, N. (1996). Ocular injuries in battered women. *Ophthalmology, 103*, 148–151.

Bergman, B., and Brismar, B. (1991). A 5-year follow-up study of 117 battered women. *American Journal of Public Health, 81*, 1486–1488.

Campbell, J.C. (1994). Child abuse and wife abuse: The connections. *Maryland Medical Journal, 43*, 349–350.

Campbell, J.C., Coben, H., McLoughlin, E., Dearwater, S., Nah, G., Glass, N., *et al.* (2001). An evaluation of a system-change training model to improve emergency department response to battered women. *Academic Emergency Medicine, 8*, 131–138.

Cascardi, M., Langhinrichsen, J., and Vivian, D. (1992). Marital aggression. Impact, injury, and health correlates for husbands and wives. *Archives of Internal Medicine, 152*, 1178–1184.

Coben, J.H., Forjuoh, S.N., and Gondolf, E.W. (1999). Injuries and health care use in women with partners in batterer intervention programs. *Journal of Family Violence, 14*, 83–93.

Coker, A.L., Davis, K.E., Arias, I., Desai, S., Sanderson, M., Brandt, H.M., and Smith, P.H. (2002). Physical and mental health effects of intimate partner violence for men and women. *American Journal of Preventive Medicine, 23*, 260–268.

Dutton, M.A., Mitchell, B., and Haywood, Y. (1996). The emergency department as a violence prevention center. *Journal of the American Medical Women's Association, 51*, 92–117.

Edleson J.L. (2000). Children's witnessing of adult domestic violence. *Journal of Interpersonal Violence, 14*, 839–870.

Fanslow, J.L., Norton, R.N., and Robinson, E.M. (1999). One-year follow-up of an emergency department protocol for abused women. *Australian and New Zealand Journal of Public Health, 23*, 418–420.

Fanslow, J.L., Norton, R., Robinson, E.M., and Spinola, C. (1998). Outcome evaluation of an emergency department protocol of care of partner abuse. *Australian and New Zealand Journal of Public Health, 22*, 598–603.

Gleason, W. (1993). Mental disorders in battered women: An empirical study. *Violence and Victims, 8*, 53–68.

Hamberger, L.K., and Ambuel, B. (2000). Community collaboration to develop research programs in partner violence. *Journal of Aggression, Maltreatment, and Trauma, 4*, 239–272.

Hamberger, L.K., and Patel, D. (2004). Why health-care professionals are reluctant to intervene in cases of ongoing domestic abuse. In K.A. Kendall-Tackett (ed.), *Health consequences of abuse in the family: A clinical guide for evidence-based practice* (pp. 63–80). Washington, DC: American Psychological Association.

Hamberger, L.K., and Phelan, M.B. (2004). *Domestic violence screening and intervention in medical and mental health settings: Research and practice.* New York: Springer.

Hamberger, L.K., Saunders, D.G., and Hovey, M. (1992). Prevalence of domestic violence in community practice and rate of physician inquiry. *Family Medicine, 24,* 83–287.

Hamberger, L.K., Ambuel, B., Marbella, A., and Donze, J. (1998). Physician interaction with battered women. The women's perspective. *Archives of Family Medicine, 7,* 575–582.

Hamberger, L.K., Guse, C., Boerger, J., Minsky, D., Pape, D., and Folsom, C. (2004). Evaluation of a healthcare provider training program to identify and help partner violence victims. *Journal of Family Violence, 19,* 1–11.

Hartzell, K.N., Botek, A.A., and Goldberg, S.H. (1996). Orbital fractures in women due to sexual assault and domestic violence. *Opthalmology, 103,* 953–957.

Harwell, T.S., Casten, R.J., Armstrong, K.A., Dempsey, S., Coons, H.L., and Davis, M. (1998). Evaluation Committee of the Philadelphia Family Violence Working Group. Results of a domestic violence training program offered to the staff of urban community health centers. *American Journal of Preventive Medicine, 15,* 235–242.

Johnson, M., and Elliott, B.A. (1997). Domestic violence among family practice patients in midsized and rural communities. *Journal of Family Practice, 44,* 391–399.

Kramer, A., Lorenzon, D., and Mueller, G. (2004). Prevalence of intimate partner violence and health implications for women using emergency departments and primary care clinics. *Women's Health Issues, 14,* 19–29.

Krasnoff, M., and Moscati, R. (2002). Domestic violence screening and referral can be effective. *Annals of Emergency Medicine, 40,* 485–492.

Kyriacou, D.N., Anglin, D., Taliaferro, E., Stone, S., Tubb, T., Linden, J.A., *et al.* (1999). Risk factors for injury to women from domestic violence. *The New England Journal of Medicine, 341,* 1892–1898.

Le, B.T., Ueeck, B., Dierks, E.J., Homer, L.D., and Potter, B.E. (2001). Maxillofacial injuries associated with domestic violence. *Journal of Oral and Maxillofacial Surgeons, 59*, 1277–1283.

McCaw B., Berman, W.H., Syme, S.L., and Hunkeler, E.F. (2001). Beyond screening for domestic violence: A systems model approach in a managed care setting. *American Journal of Preventive Medicine, 21*, 170–176.

McFarlane, J.M., Groff, J.Y., Obrien, J.A., and Watson, K. (2006). Secondary prevention of IPV: A randomized controlled trial. *Nursing Research, 55*, 52–61.

McKibben, L., DeVos, E., and Newberger, E. (1989). Victimization of mothers of abused children: A controlled study. *Pediatrics, 4*, 531–535.

McLeer, S.V., Anwar, R., Herman, S., and Maquiling, K. (1989). Education is not enough: A systems failure in protecting battered women. *Annals of Emergency Medicine, 18*, 651–653.

Minsky-Kelly, D., Hamberger, L.K., Pape, D.A., and Wolff, M. (2005). We've had training, now what? Qualitative analysis of barriers to domestic violence screening and referral in a health care setting. *Journal of Interpersonal Violence, 20*, 1288–1309.

Muelleman, R.L., and Liewer, J.D. (1998). How often do women in the emergency department without intimate violence injuries return with such injuries? *Academic Emergency Medicine, 5*, 982–985.

Muelleman, R.L., Lenaghan, P.A., and Pakeiser, R.A. (1998). Non-battering presentations to the ED of women in physically abusive relationships. *American Journal of Emergency Medicine, 16*, 128–131.

Nicolaides, C. (1999). *Voices of survivors*. San Francisco, CA: Family Violence Prevention Fund.

Perciaccante, V.J., Ochs, H.A., and Dodson, T.B. (1999). Head, neck, and facial injuries as markers of domestic violence in women. *Journal of Oral and Maxillofacial Surgery, 57*, 760–762.

Rath, G.D., Jarratt, L.G., and Leonardson, G. (1989). Rates of domestic violence against adult women by men partners. *Journal of the American Board of Family Practice, 2*, 227–233.

Rennison, C.M., and Welshers, S. (2000). *Bureau of Justice Statistics special report on intimate partner violence*. Washington, DC: National Institute of Justice.

Rodriguez, M.A., Quiroga, S.S., and Bauer, H.M. (1996). Breaking the silence:

Battered women's perspectives on medical care. *Archives of Family Medicine, 5*, 153–158.

Rodriguez, M.A., Bauer, H.M., McLoughlin, E., and Grumbach, K. (1999). Screening and intervention for intimate partner abuse practices and attitudes of primary care physicians. *Journal of the American Medical Association, 282*, 468–474.

Saunders, D.G., Hamberger, L.K., and Hovey, M. (1993). Indicators of woman abuse based on a chart review at a family practice center. *Archives of Family Medicine, 2*, 537–543.

Stark, E., and Flitcraft, A.H. (1988). Women and children at risk: A feminist perspective on child abuse. *International Journal of Health Services, 18*, 97–119.

Stark, E., and Flitcraft, A. (1995). Killing the beast within: Woman battering and suicidality. *International Journal of Health Services, 25*, 43–64.

Sugg, N.K., and Inui, T. (1992). Primary care physicians' response to domestic violence: Opening Pandora's Box. *Journal of the American Medical Association, 267*, 3157–3160.

Thompson, R.S., Rivara, F.P., Thompson, D.C., Barlow, W.E., Sugg, N.K., Maiuro, R.D., and Rubanowice, D.M. (2000). Identification and management of domestic violence. A randomized trial. *American Journal of Preventive Medicine, 19*, 253–263.

Wagner, P.J., and Mongan, P.F. (1998). Validating the concept of abuse. Women's perceptions of defining behaviors and the effects of emotional abuse on health indicators. *Archives of Family Medicine, 7*, 25–29.

Warshaw, C. (1996). Domestic violence: Changing theory, changing practice. *Journal of the American Women's Medical Association, 51*, 87–92.

Wisconsin Department of Health and Family Services. *Healthiest Wisconsin 2010: A Partnership Plan to Improve the Health of the Public*. Madison, Wisconsin.

World Health Organization (1996). *WHO global consultation on violence and health. Violence: A public health priority* (Document WHO/EHA/SPI.POA.2.s). Geneva: World Health Organization.

Author index

Subject index